Living with Certainty™
EVERYDAY SPIRITUALITY

Copyright © 2010 Kristi LeBlanc

All rights reserved.

Printed and bound in the United States of America.
ISBN 978-0-9843818-0-7

Published by Thundersnow Publishing
14405 West Colfax Avenue, Lakewood, CO 80401
First printing in 2010 by Thundersnow Publishing LLC

Without limiting the rights under copyright reserved above, no part of this publication may be reproduced in or introduced into a retrieval system, or transmitted, in any form or by any means (electronic, mechanical, photocopying, recording, or by an information storage and retrieval system)—except by a reviewer who may quote brief passages in a review to be printed in a magazine, newspaper, or on the Internet—without the prior written permission of both the copyright owner and publisher of this book.

Although the author and publisher have made every effort to ensure the accuracy and completeness of information contained in this book, we assume no responsibility for errors, inaccuracies, omissions, or any inconsistency herein. Any slights of people, places, or organizations are unintentional.

The scanning, uploading, and distribution of this book via the Internet or via any other means without the permission of the publisher is illegal and punishable by law. Please purchase only authorized, electronic editions and do not participate in or encourage electronic piracy of copyrightable materials. Your support of the author's rights is appreciated.

Living with Certainty

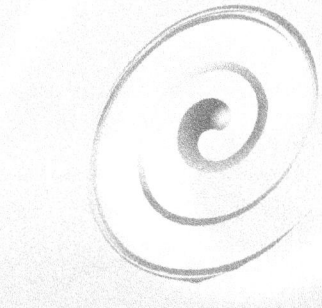

Experience Deep-Soul JOY

authenticity   spirituality   discovery

Kristi LeBlanc

Founder & CEO, Living with Certainty, LLC™

*Dedicated to the loves of my life—
Chase, Alexa, Kit, and CJ*

*We are such a blessed and happy family.
You each make me so proud.
May you always live lives of deep-soul joy.
44 Infinity*

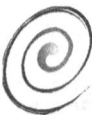

"Words are things, and a small drop of ink falling like dew upon a thought, produces that which makes thousands, perhaps millions, think."
—Sir Aubrey De Vere

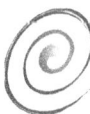

Table of Contents

Acknowledgments — xi
Introduction — xiii

PART I
The Living with Certainty Philosophy
1

Chapter 1: Hard, but Happy Work — 2
Chapter 2: Your Deep-Soul Joy — 7
Chapter 3: Your Spiritual Power Frequency — 12
Chapter 4: Signs, Signals, Symbols, and Synchronicities — 21
Chapter 5: Static — 32

PART II
Discovering the Life the Universe Always Intended for You to Live
39

Chapter 6: Your Inspired Soul-View — 40
Chapter 7: Awareness — 50
Chapter 8: Universal Interconnectivity — 56
Chapter 9: Meditation — 64
Chapter 10: Your Purpose and Purposeful Authenticity — 69
Chapter 11: Your Internal Instruction System — 83
Chapter 12: Inspiration and Creativity — 91

PART III
The Living with Certainty Lifestyle: The Energy Enablers
97

Chapter 13: Spiritual Energy — 100
Love • Self-Awareness and Self-Love • Compassion • Service • Allowance and Surrender • Revelation and Enlightenment • Acceptance • Prayer • Peace • Silence and Solitude • Communing with Nature

Chapter 14: Mind and Thoughts — 121
Morality • Honesty, Truth, and Facts • Intention • Openness • Clarity • Choice • Fear, Courage, and Confidence • Affirmations • Kindness and Tolerance • Optimism • The Law of Attraction

Chapter 15: Actions — 144
Risks and Leaps of Faith • Effort and Excellence • Commitment, Persistence, and Perseverance • Change • Learning • Deceleration and Balance • Simplicity • Goal-Setting and Planning • Responsibility • Well-Being • Karma • Using Luck • Journals and Writing • Travel and Exploration

Chapter 16: Relationships — 163
Family and Teaching the World's Children • Teachers and Wise Counsel • Personal Power • Harm No One • Your Ancestors • Boundaries • Pets

Chapter 17: Beliefs — 177
Conscious and Subconscious Beliefs • Faith and Trust • Limitless Abundance and Your Dreams • Receptivity • Visualization • Hope • Convictions • Expectations

Chapter 18: Gratitude — 188
Appreciation • Count Your Blessings Every Day • Grace and Reverence • Celebrations • Giving and Generosity • Rituals • Honor and Commemoration

Chapter 19: Progress — 196
Legacy • Endurance • Evolution, Transformation, and Becoming • Patience • Prioritization • Humor • Freedom

PART IV
What's Holding You Back?
203

Chapter 20: Ego	204
Chapter 21: Negative Thoughts	211
Chapter 22: Conditioning	216
Chapter 23: Failure and Regret	219
Chapter 24: Adversity and Problem Solving	224
Chapter 25: Criticism	228
Chapter 26: Measuring Up	234
Chapter 27: Forgiveness	239
Chapter 28: Doubt	243
Chapter 29: Denial	244
Chapter 30: Skeptics	246
Epilogue	*249*
Endnotes	*255*
Recommended Reading	*258*
About the Author	*260*

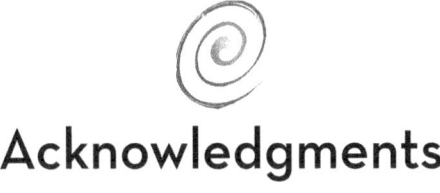

Acknowledgments

MY SINCERE THANKS to everyone who helped me bring *Living with Certainty* to life.

To Chase, my best friend and soul mate, for flying cover for me nights, weekends, and basically around the clock in order for me to follow my inspiration. Your contributions, as well as your support and belief in me, my vision, and the Living with Certainty philosophy were essential, and I am completely indebted to you. It took immense patience and love for you to read with such care and contribute to so many versions of unedited manuscripts. You saved me from making many errors.

To GiGi, my beloved mother, for providing so much loving help and support, particularly with the kids, so that I could focus on my work.

To Kevin Quinn, my dear friend, for believing in my vision and supporting and advising me along my journey.

To Sharon Goldinger for understanding my vision and helping me to create the overall structure for *Living with Certainty*. To Debra Bokur for your enthusiasm and wonderful ability to scale down the manuscript while at the same time adding so much through your skillful editing. And to Dan Forrest-Bank for contributing your impressive creative and design abilities to the brand logo, cover, and layout.

And to my three precious children for driving me to complete this project faster than I ever would have if not for your repeated question—"How much longer?" Lexy, you are magic and you inspire me to be the best I can be.

Introduction

"If you develop the absolute sense of certainty that powerful beliefs provide, then you can get yourself to accomplish virtually anything, including those things that other people are certain are impossible."
—William Lyon Phelps

TIME AND AGAIN, we've heard "experts" dispense the same old theoretical advice—*Do what you love and success (and money) will follow.* Yet, developing awareness of your passions, defining success, devising a strategy, and taking productive action every day is often easier said than done. It requires specific understanding, guidance, discipline, and effort. The good news is that you have everything you need—here, now, today—to begin. All that's required is that you discover your *inspired soul-view* and learn to listen to and trust in the natural, hard-wired guidance system that already exists within you. I call this collection of feelings, emotions, instinct, and intuition your *internal instruction system.* Through *Living with Certainty,* I will teach you how to access this resource.

The entire premise of this book is that irrespective of your place in life today, you are capable of experiencing great joy while learning to harness and elevate your personal energy in the quest to discover—and share—your greatest gifts with the world. We are all intended to be vibrant, energetic forces in the co-creation of our lives. While we clearly don't have complete control over every aspect of our lives, we must deliberately and proactively take action and move in alignment with our inspired soul-view and the guidance we receive from Source energy through hunch, instinct, intuition, or old-fashioned gut feelings. The most successful, joyous, self-actualized people share this trait: they are aware of, and in tune with, every aspect of their personal energy and understand the significance it plays in the co-creation of their purposeful lives.

Purposeful Authenticity and Work

I've learned much about spirituality throughout my career in business consulting. You may think business and spirituality to be a strange combination. However, our careers are an intrinsic part of our lives, and should be interconnected with our essence. To take this concept a step further, our livelihoods should be aligned with our soul's Earthly purpose if we're to experience lasting joy and fulfillment. Your occupation was never intended to be solely a paycheck, or an avenue to power or prominence. Certainly, you don't want to spend your days toiling away at an activity you dislike. No one does. Rather, your life's work should be an expression of *purposeful authenticity* that allows you to experience personal joy, growth, and enlightenment while also serving the universe in an inimitable way. Your work takes up most of your waking hours, so it's essential that you spend your time expressing your natural passions and aptitudes.

Through thousands of conversations, I consistently observed vast differences in people relative to feelings of success and failure, joy and pain, and fulfillment and frustration. *Who am I? ... What do I really have to offer? ... How can I get more joy and satisfaction from my job? ... Why isn't this working for me? ... What should I really be doing? ... How can I make a more significant contribution? How can I make more money?* To my surprise, while roughly half of the individuals I met were extremely content, purpose-driven, and fulfilled, the other half with similar wealth and positional power were completely disenchanted and distraught over their career and life paths. Although the majority of these executives were equally polished and accomplished, the truly fulfilled and passionate people had a higher level of energy, originality, enthusiasm, and spark.

By studying these outwardly successful people, the following points became obvious: 1) success is relative and you must define what it means to you, never accepting someone else's definition, and 2) your personal sense of achievement and success comes only from the extent to which you experience joy and fulfillment in your life. Over time, I discovered that the essential difference was that the fulfilled individuals were expressing and satisfying their soul's purpose and authenticity. They innately knew how to empower themselves through the daily—and even moment-to-moment—application of enlightened life skills that supported the expression of their purposeful authenticity. This naturally led to the experience of their *deep-soul joy*.

It became clear to me that we must all begin more deeply contemplating our lives and how we spend our time. We must consciously choose our "work" only after much deliberation, discussion, and thought from a far broader and deeper perspective than our current process. Over time, I developed my Living with Certainty philosophy and began to share with others this practical spiritual solution to daily life, including career management, with the goal of simplifying the achievement of purposeful authenticity, fulfillment, and deep-soul joy.

Even if you choose for one reason or another not to have a career, you must decide how you are going to express your purposeful authenticity. It is our work—including parenting, hobbies, and service—that allows us to express our Earthly purpose and to experience self-actualization.

If the word "work" carries a negative connotation for you, it's a sure sign that you've not yet aligned your work with your soul's Earthly purpose. You cannot be at your happiest and most fulfilled when your work requires that you leave behind your joy, authenticity, creativity, and talents. When you figure out how to articulate your purposeful authenticity in your work, you're expressing the aspect of your self and soul that is intended to be developed, shared, and explored in your Earthly life. Further, you are naturally contributing in uniquely original and purposeful ways that allow you to experience a purposeful, fulfilling, and joyous life path—*the life the universe always intended for you to live.*

Exploring Your Self and Soul
While life in our universe is indubitably mysterious and profound,

it's clear to me that our Earthly journeys are intended for exploring ourselves and our souls, not merely for accumulating possessions, or being perpetually battered as if living through a torrential storm. Your life's adventure should unquestionably include discovering your various dimensions, including your purpose, potentiality, and passions. The essential first step is to open your mind and awareness to the notion that you are spirit as well as mind and body, and to initiate the revelation of your inspired soul-view. This is the 360-degree, panoramic view of the life your soul entered into Earthly physicality to experience. Think of it as the profound, unspoken, innermost inspiration that fills your awareness with authenticity, inspiration, and purpose. Your direction for full participation in a life that expresses your purposeful authenticity will become clear. You can and will create profound and joyful change in your life.

Isn't the Universe Fundamentally Uncertain?

First of all, what does it mean to *"live with certainty" in a fundamentally uncertain universe?* It means that you live daily in a way that expresses your inspired soul-view and purposeful authenticity. It means that your emotions and instinct guide you toward a life of passion, joy, purpose, love, service, and compassion. You are certain when you feel good, purposeful, and fulfilled; when your instinct and intuition speak to you; when a sign or synchronous event appears for you; when your vibrational frequency is heightened or lowered; and above all, when you are experiencing deep-soul joy.

This approach reinforces the internal certainty that you're making the right decisions and taking the right *actions*. Your internal instruction system, when fully in tune with *Source energy* (the ever-flowing, all-knowing creative energy of the universe through which we are all interconnected and from which all Earthly physicality emanates) and your inspired soul-view, enables brilliant boldness and authenticity over your actions. One of life's most important tasks is to uncover what's right for you at your individual emotional and soul level. The energy of certainty feels good and right. We only feel truly good, joyous, fulfilled, and peaceful when we act in fundamentally loving, compassionate, and inspired soul-view-aligned ways. These are high-vibrational frequency states. This is precisely how we live with certainty.

Life Through a Spiritual Lens

Everything in our universe is composed of energy—from our thoughts, feelings, and words, to the chair in which you're sitting. Until we learn to understand, purify, and heighten our own personal energy vibrations, we will continue to experience disharmony, anxiety, fear, insecurity, and internal uncertainty in our lives. This is far from being a new concept. For centuries, the ancient Chinese concept of Qi (chi) has recognized that every aspect of the universe is comprised of an all-powerful, intelligent energy force. Reiki, the centuries-old Japanese technique for healing, relaxation, and stress reduction, maintains that "life force energy" flows through us, keeping us alive. The Chakra system, a concept documented for the first time in the Hindu scriptures known as the Upanishads (1200–900 B.C.), refers to seven major force centers, or chakras, in the human body which serve as focal points for the reception and transmission of energies.

Living with Certainty takes this ancient knowledge and helps you to understand and naturally heighten your energy vibrations, teaching you to think, believe, and act in ways that encourage and improve your life. By learning to create balance and harmony between your mind, body, and spirit, you naturally become skilled at sending energy out to the universe at a high-vibrating frequency. Life becomes easier, unforced, natural, and flowing when you live with certainty.

When you live *without* certainty, it's difficult to experience the flow of your *spiritual power frequency*, because you don't vibrate energy at the optimal frequency level required for alignment with the flow of Source energy. While you may be able to find financial or material success, it's unlikely that you will experience the fulfillment and deep-soul joy that comes from living a life in expression of your purposeful authenticity.

Living with Certainty allows you to recognize and act upon the affirming and guiding signs, signals, symbols, and synchronous events that emanate from Source energy, helping you to remain powerfully in the flow of your spiritual power frequency. These signs and synchronicities affirm your path and allow you to co-create and shape your life in alignment with your inspired soul-view.

About This Book

Living with Certainty is designed to be a guide to help you align with the flow your spiritual power frequency. When you live with certainty, your energy essence will vibrate at a high, pure level. Your instincts will be aligned and strong. Signs, signals, symbols, and synchronicities will poke, prod, and guide you along your intended life path. This approach to life will allow you to discover your authentic, deep-soul joy through the following:

- Dwelling in awareness of the present moment and sensing your interconnectivity with all else
- Discovering your inspired soul-view and purposeful authenticity
- Moving through daily life resonating high-frequency energy vibrations through actions, thoughts, feelings, beliefs, relationships, and gratitude in accordance with the 65 "Energy Enablers"
- Aligning with the flow of your spiritual power frequency
- Eliminating negative, static-inducing thoughts, beliefs, relationships, and actions from your daily life that can negate alignment with your spiritual power frequency and purposeful authenticity
- Being spiritually deliberate and focused in your thoughts, actions, beliefs, relationships, and expressions of gratitude
- Listening to and acting upon your emotions, hunches, instinct, and intuition (your internal instruction system)
- Following the guidance of signs, signals, symbols, and synchronicities

- Relieving yourself of the exhausting pressure of an ego-centered, hollow grab for material trophies

This book provides simple, time-tested, and practical guidance that can be incorporated into your daily life. When you are exhausted and frustrated from toiling away without moving forward or experiencing any joy, Living with Certainty can transition you out of your rut, moving you ever closer to experiencing deep-soul joy and the life the universe always intended for you to live.

The first half of the book is informational, while the latter half is comprised of the Living with Certainty Energy Enablers, traits possessed by the most authentic, joyous, and purposeful individuals. I conclude the book with the section "What's Holding You Back?", a discussion of commonly encountered, problematic areas that create static, lower your vibrational frequency, and thwart your efforts to live with certainty.

Energy Enablers Create the Optimal Energy Environment

The 65 Living with Certainty Energy Enablers serve as techniques and tools to focus, heighten, and intensify your everyday energy vibrations. Many of the Energy Enablers are traits, skills, activities, attributes, and approaches that are already a part of your personality and daily experience, though you may not be practicing them in a way that consistently raises your vibrational frequency. As you make the choice to live a spiritual life of certainty, the Energy Enablers will help you to live a life of heightened, pure energy vibration.

Spirituality as Lifestyle

A true spiritual journey is a lifestyle—part and parcel of everything you do on a daily basis. Living with Certainty provides a practical spiritual foundation—a deliberate way to approach and align your thoughts, emotions, beliefs, relationships, and actions. The process allows plenty of room for personal choice and authenticity as you carve out a unique life path in partnership with your inspired soul-view, and seamlessly learn to blend the various facets of your Earthly life with Source energy.

This isn't a process that should be undertaken only when you want or need something but is a belief system so deep and intrinsic to your ongoing growth and spiritual development that you cannot live any other way. It's the ultimate way of honoring your self, your soul, your life, and your contribution to the universe.

Over time, Living with Certainty will become your dominant nature, further defining who you are and how you live as you absorb and practice the 65 Energy Enablers. Once this becomes your approach to life, Source energy responds to you—not with gifts, but with guidance. Once this power is understood and ingrained deep within you, it can never be taken away.

So, my friend, as you read on, take heart. This abundant universe can manifest far greater things than you can ever imagine for yourself. It's never too late. Keep an open mind. Believe. Have confidence in your ability to discover and express your purposeful authenticity and to manifest the life the universe always intended for you to live. And then get ready—here come the best days of your life.

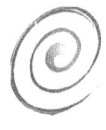

PART I
The Living with Certainty Philosophy

"Re-examine all you have been told … . Dismiss what insults your soul."
—Walt Whitman

To begin your Living with Certainty journey, you must first consider and embrace certain ideas. For example, humans are first and foremost souls, which are the essence of our physical beings—who we *really* are. Our souls enter into Earthly physicality in order to express our purposeful authenticity and experience deep-soul joy. Within us already dwells the requisite power and resources for an extraordinarily fulfilled existence.

We're hardwired with an internal instruction system that serves to guide us in alignment with our inspired soul-view through instinct, feeling, and intuition. Signs, signals, symbols, and synchronicities are communication from Source energy that grace us with guidance.

This all-encompassing, powerful, unseen energy plane surrounds us and allows us to co-create our Earthly lives. Our actions, beliefs, feelings, and thoughts create energetic vibrations that interact with, and respond to, Source energy. Through heightened awareness and diligence we can align with this flow. Without question, you possess the power to co-create the life the universe always intended for you to live in tandem with Source energy. Source energy loves you and awaits your individual connection.

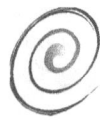

CHAPTER 1

Hard, but Happy Work

"You are like a poor man who doesn't realize he lives on top of buried treasure. The earth of body, mind, and speech obscures the fact that you are already enlightened and keeps you impoverished by the sufferings of life."
—Kunkhyen Longchen Rabjam

AT THIS VERY MOMENT, everything you need to begin real transformation dwells inside of you. This is the time to stop, think, believe, and behave your way out of what may feel like an empty life. By undertaking the Living with Certainty approach, you're giving yourself the gift of exploring new possibilities for living an authentic life.

Like many people, you may have explored numerous self-help methods in search of the one big breakthrough that would finally end your anxiety, emptiness, pain, and restlessness. You may feel as though you've tried everything without ever moving forward. Maybe, despite having achieved status, success, and financial freedom, you still feel incomplete. Deep inside, you know one thing for sure: this is not the life you are meant to live.

We're All in This Together

You're not alone. Your feelings are far more common and widespread than you may have guessed. People of all ages, backgrounds, incomes, and nationalities suffer from a profound lack of fulfillment, purpose, and joy. They, like you, have worked hard chasing the American dream, only to wake up asking, *What happened? This isn't how I thought my life would end up.*

Does any of the following sound familiar?

- You know you're capable of more, yet your current existence

Chapter 1: Hard, but Happy Work

feels just ordinary.
- You long for relief from daily pressures, fears, and insecurities.
- You feel lonely, restless, or trapped, not knowing where or how you fit in.
- You don't know the way out, but you are willing to commit to discovering a new path before you run out of time.

Leaving Your Comfort Zone

Consider yourself forewarned: Much work lies ahead—hard, but happy work. Your quest to discover deep-soul joy won't be successful if you merely deposit artificial layers of emotions on top of your pain and discontent. You'll need commitment, discipline, self-control, and persistence to dissolve the old habits, behaviors, and patterns accumulated over a lifetime. New, raw feelings will emerge that will need to be processed. This journey can be challenging and difficult because as you undertake living with certainty, you will increasingly develop an awareness of events, circumstances, and relationships that bring you pain and confliction. This is an essential part of your journey, for only then can you begin to figure out why you feel the way you do. You must make peace with these feelings once and for all.

Much time and effort are required when undertaking an authentic spiritual journey if it's to result in the release of your spirit's innate wisdom regarding your Earthly purpose. Though Living with Certainty is a practical approach intended to be integrated into your daily life, enormous commitment, discipline, and patience are still required. An essential aspect of the Living with Certainty journey is patience, and allowing yourself the necessary time to release your demons and experience real growth. This isn't an instantaneous spiritual makeover, but a process that unfolds naturally and differently for everyone. The fact that you're reading this book indicates that you are ready to begin the required work.

Take a moment, right now, to ask yourself this question: *Am I ready to break free of the shackles of my ego, and the other aspects of Earthly physicality preventing me from bringing the power of*

Source energy fully into my life? Next, ask yourself this: *Am I willing and open to examining every aspect of myself?* You cannot begin to change your outer life without first doing the obligatory inner work. For some, little inner work is required; for others, a lifetime of ongoing inner work may be necessary. We all have the same capacity to co-create the life the universe always intended for us to live, it's just that some of us have more work to do to discover our inspired soul-view, release our baggage, and heal old wounds.

Attention Required

You're probably wondering what, exactly, is this potential *hard work?* Anyone who's starving for wisdom, fulfillment, and deep-soul joy will likely need to expend some level of attention, effort, and discipline—be it assessment, contemplation, healing, release, or centering. The work begins with accepting yourself as you are today, and may also include:

- Discovering and resolving underlying issues to access the root of your pain
- Taking a hard look at conditioning and beliefs that can block your progress
- Facing down painful feelings in order to experience and understand them

This process takes time, patience, faith, and self-love. Living with certainty requires that you discover the root causes of your blockages, baggage, pain, and suffering; you must allow yourself to fully experience the emotion, and not just deal with the symptoms. Foundational problems never miraculously disappear without work. *The Living with Certainty Discovery Guide* will help you to begin to ask yourself the right questions, and help you to examine issues that you've had for years.

Before we go any further, it should be understood that the approach outlined in this book is not intended to replace any therapy that may be needed to help you heal and move forward; it is not intended to cure mental or physical illness. If you suffer, or have suffered, from depression, abuse, catastrophes, traumatic events, or psychosis, you should seek appropriate professional psychological counseling.

Peeling Back the Layers

In order to arouse, stir, and awaken the healthy "real" you, you must allow yourself to lean into feelings of discomfort and pain rather than shut them down or deny them. Think of this process as slowly peeling the layers from an onion until you finally reach its innermost heart. This takes courage, but the more layers of baggage, life-long conditioning, and ego-personality that you peel away, the more you'll experience your true essence and authenticity. By allowing yourself to experience and explore these emotions as they arise, you can begin to lessen their stranglehold on you. As you peel away layers of ego, the negative voices, limiting perceptions, and false impressions in your head—everything that stands between you and your inspired soul-view—will begin to fade. Visualize this process as bringing your pain into the light that shines from deep within you.

Steel yourself to endure whatever painful emotions surface, allowing yourself to feel them fully. If you run from them or ignore them, they will never go away. They'll just lie in wait, eventually surfacing and undoing all of your efforts. Over time, after you lean into the pain again and again, it lessens. You start to let go of it; you begin to get over it. It's no longer there, hiding in the shadows. Through this courageous work, you will nurture and promote your own spiritual awakening.

The Never-Ending Journey

Living with Certainty is a journey comprised of your life's most purposeful and rewarding work. Every step you take as you live with certainty is a positive step in the right direction. The reality, however, is that you will encounter bumps along the way. This is the nature of Earthly life, and necessary to the process of discovering inner peace, purpose, strength, and freedom.

This journey is about much more than monetary and material

accumulation. You *already* exist in beautiful completeness at the most fundamental level, your essence. As one of your deepest commitments and intentions, Living with Certainty puts the responsibility for your life squarely on you, designating you as the source of power, not the victim. This requires the creation of an optimal inner landscape where room exists for you to engage in new spiritual and mental activities.

As you master Living with Certainty, you'll see that there is no endgame. This journey reflects the ongoing purpose of your life, where you will continually discover new aspects of your inspired soul-view and achieve new levels of deep-soul joy. Your journey will only become more fascinating along the way, and more intense as you experience deeper levels of your spiritual existence.

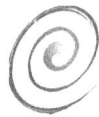

CHAPTER 2

Your Deep-Soul Joy

*"Suddenly I realize
That if I stepped out of my body I would break
Into blossom."*
—James Wright

ARISTOTLE PUT IT BEST when he wrote, "Happiness is the meaning and the purpose of life, the whole aim and end of human existence." We are all hardwired spiritually and psychologically to pursue joy and pleasure, two of our core motivations in life. The pursuit of joy itself renders a more purposeful life, yet real joy and happiness remain elusive for so many of us. As you live with certainty, aligning your thoughts, actions, and beliefs with your inspired soul-view and purposeful authenticity, you open the door to deep-soul joy. It doesn't matter who or where you are. The power resides within you now to live a life of deep-soul joy. Within your intention to undertake this journey to joy lies purpose and power.

What Is Deep-Soul Joy?

Deep-soul joy results from living a life that expresses your purposeful authenticity and is in complete alignment with your inspired soul-view. This joyous state of Being is experienced as your soul is freed to blossom into its natural state. As your essence becomes aligned with, and fully enveloped in, Source energy's universal love, you internally experience the powerful and affirming energy of the spiritual realm. Deep-soul joy is dependent upon nothing external or material. It is a gift to us, an affirmation that we're living the life the universe always intended for us to live.

When it is the ongoing baseline of your Earthly existence, the profoundly peaceful state of deep-soul joy also holds super-charged moments that cause you to feel extraordinarily alive, vibrant, and aware of your innate connection to Source energy. Sensations of energetic euphoria and intense feelings of awe and gratitude pulse through your being as your awareness heightens of the extraordinary opportunity Earthly physicality has provided you to explore and express your potential and your purposeful authenticity. Deep-soul joy is many things, namely the following:

- The unmistakable, powerful, rising emergence of your soul's energetic perfection into your awareness as your mind-body-spirit merge in affirming, complete alignment with that moment's Earthly existence
- Affirmation that you are living a life that energetically aligns with and expresses your inspired soul-view and purposeful authenticity
- A palpable, energetic connection with Source energy
- Profound awareness of the here and now, along with a deep sense of being in the right place at the right time
- Deep peacefulness, fulfillment, and joy from knowing that you're living out your Earthly purpose while fully realizing your aptitudes and abilities
- Recognition that you are in the optimal, high-vibrational energetic environment to co-create your soul's Earthly dreams, the life the universe always intended for you to live
- Heightened awareness of every aspect of your life in each moment, and deep-felt gratitude for the inherent soul-developing nature of all of your life's circumstances
- A strong sense of hope, faith, optimism, and personal power
- An openness and receptiveness to powerfully flowing Source energy
- A feeling of liberation and boundlessness as you revel in the transformational power of joy and experience your soul at the deepest, most profound level

Deep-soul joy provides proof and reassurance that we needn't be tethered to suffering. Once you live from your soul and align with your purposeful authenticity, your perspective broadens and attaches deeper meaning to everything you do and everything that happens to you. You become infused with natural, effortless gratitude, hope, love, and reverence for every aspect of your life. Even in the midst of chaos, you remain centered in this continual, everlasting core of comfort, peace, and joy.

Deep-Soul Joy Requires Heightened Awareness

Deep-soul joy requires that you live fully in the present moment—there is no deep-soul joy in the past or future. Just being in an inspired, perfect, harmonious moment provides supreme fulfillment. It may often seem that everyone around you is constantly complaining while you have a perpetual song in your heart.

Deep-Soul Joy Requires Purposeful Authenticity

Experiencing your deep-soul joy requires the intentional and active pursuit of your inspired soul-view. Your greatest joy will emanate through the expression of your soul-view's purposeful authenticity and its accompanying freedom, fulfillment, inspiration, and connectivity. Life will become smoother and more joyous as you begin to experience increasing levels of love and support that flow directly into your life.

What Deep-Soul Joy Is Not

Deep-soul joy does not require that you waste your time by blindly pursuing people, circumstances, or material possessions that produce fleeting sensations of pleasure or gratification. Happiness is flimsy; deep-soul joy lives in your core.

Up until now, you may only have known transitory moments of surface happiness based upon external situations or possessions, while your inner-being remained in turmoil and flux. Illusions of momentary happiness can easily be created through entertainment, pleasurable external circumstances, or material possessions.

Surface happiness doesn't last. Deep-soul joy, however, isn't a fleeting positive experience, emotion, good mood, or pleasurable time. Rather, it is a spiritual state that transcends whatever else is going on. Once you experience deep-soul joy, it will become your mindset—an approach to life that comes from directly experiencing your connection with Source energy. After one taste, deep-soul joy becomes a limitless well to which you'll return to drink from for the rest of your life.

A Joyous Leap of Faith

Your most significant power rests in your awareness of the manner in which your *soul* reacts to external events, and how you in turn respond physically and emotionally. Tenderness and patience are required as you journey to deep-soul joy. Soul-based spirituality cannot be forced. You may feel that you've been holding your breath till now—waiting for the big break, waiting to be exposed, waiting for an answer, waiting for some anxiety to end. Living with certainty, however, requires you to surrender and exhale. This entails a leap of faith—but if you follow your guided feelings, you'll discover a life that expresses your purposeful authenticity, and deep-soul joy naturally follows.

Joy and Genetics

We've established that deep-soul joy is not just a choice or resolution, and that hard work may be required to achieve it. You may have to reprogram yourself and create new habits, patterns, and beliefs. This takes discipline, focus, time, and effort. Research suggests that human genetics also contributes to our ability to experience happiness. In 1996, professor of psychology David Lykken and associate professor Auke Tellegen of the University of Minnesota conducted a study on the heritability of happiness, revealing that we are born with a genetic happiness baseline to which we consistently revert. Attempting to be happier than your baseline dictates can be difficult, but not impossible. If you're willing to make the inner changes needed to increase your happiness, your genetic predisposition can be overruled. More commonly, however, people prefer to make the easier changes to their external situation, rather than put forth the necessary effort for internal change—thus keeping long-lasting joy at bay.[1]

While genetics do play a role in our overall level of happiness, our thoughts, feelings, beliefs, and actions are significant as well. You may be surprised to learn that achievements, circumstances, and material possessions have little effect on joy. If you place your focus on discovering your purposeful authenticity and become engaged in the passionate expression of what you love, your inner life and happiness level would, indeed, change. Happiness and joy have everything to do with personal fulfillment. Once we all understand that deep-soul joy is possible for all of us, we can transform our world, one person at a time.

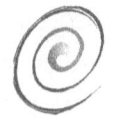

CHAPTER 3

Your Spiritual Power Frequency

*"Man is a stream whose source is hidden.
Our being is descending into us from we know not whence."*
—Ralph Waldo Emerson

CONSIDER FOR A MOMENT the concept of Qi. This ancient Chinese word is used to describe the natural, metaphysical, powerful, and pervasive energy of the universe. This concept maintains that every aspect of the universe, including humans, is made of and infused with this vital energy power. Harmony and alignment are key aspects of Qi. Negativity, problems, or discord in any facet of your life are signals that your energy is out of alignment—and, as a result, you're experiencing disharmony.

Reiki, a centuries-old Japanese technique for healing that's administered through gentle touch maintains that "life force energy" flows through us all. The word Reiki actually consists of two Japanese words—Rei, meaning "God's Wisdom or the Higher Power," and Ki, which means "life force energy." When our life force energy is low, we're more likely to feel sick or stressed; when it's high, however, we feel healthy and filled with joy.

So it goes with *spiritual power frequency*. When your mind, body, and spirit are out of balance in any way, the flow of high-frequency energy is disrupted, making it difficult, if not impossible, to co-create and experience the life the universe always intended for you to live.

For centuries, the most enlightened members of the human race have understood and maintained that an innate aspect of our soul is the ability to manifest its desires in Earthly physicality. This ability, however, remains untapped and unleveraged by many people, particularly in

American society. Instead, we've been taught to rely upon our mental and physical abilities—rather than spiritual, soul-based ones—to sustain ourselves. Sadly, this is a missed opportunity. There's so much more that can be deeply experienced and made manifest, particularly with regard to our joy. In order to do so, we must understand the concept of spiritual power frequency, an important aspect of Living with Certainty, and accept and leverage our innate spiritual powers.

What Is Spiritual Power Frequency?

Spiritual power frequency is achieved through the aligned flow of high-vibrational frequency energy between you, your inspired soul-view, and Source energy. Once this alignment is accomplished through thoughts, beliefs, emotions, gratitude, and actions that support the Earthly expression of your purposeful authenticity, you will attain a powerful, creative energy exchange with the plane of all creation. This energetic connection bridges energy planes and dimensions.

As you align with your spiritual power frequency, you will receive guidance, messages, and wise insights emanating directly from Spirit. Your path and efforts will be routinely affirmed through signs, signals, symbols, and synchronicities. The affirming and guiding benefits of this energy alignment are tantamount to sitting on the right seat on the right bus heading to the right place at the right time. Life unfolds and progresses in a way that reveals your place in the interconnected web of universal energy. Seemingly disparate aspects of your life and the lives of others suddenly and fortuitously collide. Life becomes naturally easier, filled with guiding moments and unfolding with love and abundance. Events fall into place with little effort on your part, impediments and blockages vanish, and all of your efforts seem to be more productive. Life becomes increasingly dynamic, invigorating, and brimming with implication and meaning.

How It Feels to Align with the Flow of Your Spiritual Power Frequency

We live within a vast and superb energy system, and your job is to place your spirit into its flow. When you are aligned with Source energy and your spiritual power frequency, you'll know it. You'll experience a strong sense of purpose and well-being, along with a vibrant sense of inspiration, focus, and motivation. Your life will be propelled forward with your wheels greased by the universe. You will be living in sync with oneness and flow, on your way to co-creating the life the universe always intended for you to live.

You may find that at different times in your life the strength of your spiritual power frequency ebbs or flows. Sometimes events may unfold quickly, or the rate of progress may seem to slow to a halt. While the pace may change and fluctuate, have faith that positive energy is always flowing at exactly the rate that it should, so long as you are living with certainty.

How to Align with the Flow of Your Spiritual Power Frequency

We all have the ability to align with the flow of our spiritual power frequency. It doesn't require sweat or exertion, but rather is an unforced, graceful aspect of living with certainty. Here's the formula for aligning with the flow of your spiritual power frequency:

- Raise your awareness, meditate, and take the actions outlined later in these pages to discover your inspired soul-view
- Undertake and experience thoughts and actions that express your purposeful authenticity
- Practice the Energy Enablers daily to consistently produce high-frequency energy vibrations
- Remove static-producing thoughts, feelings, beliefs, and actions that only serve to lower your vibrational frequency
- Observe and follow Source energy's guidance provided through signs, signals, symbols, and synchronicities.
- Be the change you want to see
- Co-create the life the universe always intended for you to live through inspired soul-view–aligned action as directed by your internal instruction system

Raise Your Awareness to Discover Your Inspired Soul-View

Raising your awareness means living an informed life in the present moment, remaining ever-cognizant of how you feel, becoming acutely conscious of the here and now, and not contemplating the past or the future. It's through the empty space created by your awareness that your spirit will emerge. Living a life of spirituality and discovering your inspired soul-view requires perpetually tuning into your emotions and remaining aware of what deeply reverberates within your being.

It is vital that throughout this process you remain present, centered, and balanced. Whether you experience the pain of a dysfunctional relationship, disappointment when your favorite team loses, anger when a rude driver cuts you off in traffic, or distress when the stock market dips, this is life. With awareness and focus, you can learn to process life's daily travails without allowing your feelings and emotions to become unbalanced. Over time it will become your natural state to observe, discern, and process events while remaining emotionally steady and relating to negative events as the static-inducers that they are.

Experience Thoughts and Actions in Alignment with Your Inspired Soul-View

As you begin to live with certainty, your initial work will be to discover your inspired soul-view in order to enable alignment with the flow of your spiritual power frequency. Thoughts, beliefs, and emotions emanating from alignment with your soul's purposeful authenticity vibrate at a higher frequency than non-soul-view–aligned thoughts. You cannot align dense, human energy with the purest energy of the universe until you elevate your vibrational frequency by living from a place of spirit—nor can you establish a strong energetic connection with the plane of all creation when your thoughts, beliefs, or feelings are focused on non-soul-view–aligned desires.

While you play a starring role in how your life unfolds, your thoughts, feelings, and beliefs alone aren't enough by which to steer. No matter what you do or how hard you try, you can't force outcomes if they're not in alignment with your inspired soul-view. The good news is that you don't have to force anything in order to live a life of deep-soul joy. You need only to live with certainty.

Source energy has pure love for you, and wants only those things for you that have a purpose and are in your best interest. You must acknowledge that the perspective of Source energy regarding what is in your best interest may be very different at times from your own perspective, especially if you aren't living in alignment with your inspired soul-view. Source energy wants your soul to develop—and to that end, will place great challenges in front of you. Once you are living with purposeful authenticity, in alignment with your inspired soul-view, you'll recognize that every aspect of your Earthly life, including the challenges, are part and parcel of the life the universe always intended for you to live.

Practice the Energy Enablers

The spiritual plane of existence in our universe—from which all Earthly physicality manifests—is composed of energy. Your inspired soul-view and Source energy cannot communicate with you through human words. Rather, they communicate with you through the energy of your emotions, intuition, and instincts. Your thoughts, feelings, and beliefs are composed of energy and constantly communicate directly with the powerful, unseen creative realm to co-create your life.

Once you live life in alignment with your inspired soul-view, it's necessary to continually create a high-vibrational internal energy environment through your thoughts, feelings, and beliefs. Any highly emotional (positive or negative) energy attached to your thoughts and beliefs will intensify your vibrations, and play an even more powerful role in the co-creation of what will ultimately be made manifest in your life.

In other words, the "first draft" of every aspect of your life initially exists in the powerful unseen plane of existence. The energy produced through your thoughts, beliefs, and feelings determines in large measure the way in which the universe reacts to and manifests your deep-soul desires.

Chapter 3: Your Spiritual Power Frequency

We're all hard-wired to align with the flow of our spiritual power frequency through our energy vibrations. First, though, we must learn how to access the realm of high-frequency energy. This occurs when our personal energy vibrations are honed to achieve synergy with Source energy. This can be a challenge, since the familiar Earthly realm is comprised of time, space, and matter. Its energy is dense and slow moving. The energy of the Spiritual realm is lighter, and free to vibrate at a much higher frequency.

This essential, intelligent realm of Spiritual energy is the basis for all existence in the universe: Source energy. Our souls emanate or extend like "strings" from its core, and we remain perpetually connected to the spiritual realm. When we achieve optimal alignment, or synergy, between the energy that we create and the pulsing spiritual energy within our "string," we have aligned with the flow of our spiritual power frequency.

Even if it's just a faint signal, you are always vibrating energy. Your energy vibrations move higher or lower, lighter or denser, based on what is happening internally and externally. Remember that when heightened, these are the vibrations that sing through the universal web of energy, forming the blueprint for what will be manifested for you on Earth. So feeling good at an intrinsic, deep level is essential if these vibrations are to be light and joyous enough to harmonize with the universe. Reflect upon how you've felt during some of your happiest times—loving, content, grateful, authentic, purposeful, joyous, and optimistic. These feelings are a blueprint for your ideal state. The more frequently you inhabit this ideal state of being, the more powerfully you vibrate high frequency energy. In short, how you align your feelings and express your emotions is the barometer of the quality of energy you vibrate, and determines whether you will harmonize with the flow of your spiritual power frequency.

Avoid Static-Producing Blockers

Through your awareness and your intent to maintain a high vibrational frequency at all times, you must exercise discipline in your thoughts, behaviors, and reactions. There may be perfectly acceptable Earthly reasons to feel envy, rage, anxiety, or discontent—but you must recognize the spiritual derailment that occurs when you allow negative, low-vibrational energy to weaken your power frequency. You can rise above these moments by routinely assessing how you feel and utilizing your Living with Certainty tools to raise your vibrational frequency and regain spiritual equilibrium.

Follow Guidance Provided Through Signs, Signals, Symbols, and Synchronicities

Beyond the internal communication you receive from Source energy through instinct and intuition, you're also graced with external guidance and messages from the universe through signs, signals, symbols, and synchronicities. As you raise your awareness and begin to look for this communication and guidance, you will see that the universe is sending you messages constantly. As you align with the flow of your spiritual power frequency, you will find yourself experiencing uncanny synchronistic events and occurrences. Seemingly peculiar or baffling circumstances are messages from the universe. Trust in and take time to notice and contemplate these messages, as they are intended to assist in carving out your life's path.

Be the Change You Want to See

When you align with the flow of your spiritual power frequency and are affirmed and guided by signs, signals, symbols and synchronicities, it's time to give thanks for all that you are, all that you have, and all that you will be. Live from a baseline of gratitude. The energy of gratitude contains powerful vibrations that feel good and strengthen your alignment with your spiritual power frequency.

Once you are experiencing gratitude, the real secret to co-creating and manifesting your dreams is to visualize yourself already experiencing your inspired soul-view–aligned desires and the change you want to see. Let this visualization create powerful creative energy that serves to fuel and inspire your daily actions toward the achievement of your goals. Allow yourself to experience the emotional high that the achievement of these desires will create. Your emotional energy—how you deeply feel and believe—is extremely powerful. So powerful, in fact, that when aligned with Source energy and the life the universe always intended for you to live, it can play an essential role in manifesting your desires into physical reality.

Co-Create Your Life Through Your Internal Instruction System and Inspired Soul-View–Aligned Action

Inspired soul-view–aligned action is the backbone of your efforts to co-create the life the universe always intended for you to live. When you feel the urge to take action—when hunch, instinct, intuition, or old-fashioned gut feelings are propelling you in a certain direction—move in alignment with this guidance: this is inspired soul-view–aligned action. (Note: This by no means releases you from the consequences of your actions; nor is it ever permissible to stray too far afield from the laws and mores of civil society, which must be taken into consideration before you take action.)

Though you don't have complete control over your life, our universe is a participatory one and expects your contribution and involvement. To a great extent, you are responsible for your future and what you become in Earthly physicality. You are neither an observer, nor a victim of fate or circumstance. The energy of the universe is intrinsically connected to you through your soul, and this reciprocal identity allows you to tap into its intelligence through your inspired soul-view, enabling you to actively participate in the co-creation of the life the universe always intended for you to live.

Your responsibility as a co-creator means that you cannot sit on the sidelines of your life as you may have been doing up until now. You have to become certain about what you want and deliberate in your intention to co-create it. There is no fixed or predetermined script to blindly follow. Through your internal instruction system you determine your next line, next move, and next act. Your fate is not predetermined—your spiritual energy, self-determination, choice, and actions have everything to do with how your life unfolds.

Your unique purpose in Earthly physicality is to initiate and bring forth knowledge, events, services, and circumstances that wouldn't have existed without your unique effort, intellect, and inspiration. Instead of being logistically specific about how things should come together, leave those details for Source energy to figure out through its vast, interconnected web. All the while, remain open to receiving those things that will bring you development, enlightenment, and *deep-soul joy.*

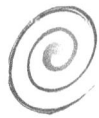

CHAPTER 4
Signs, Signals, Symbols, and Synchronicities

"There is no such thing as chance; and what seems to us merest accident springs from the deepest source of destiny."
—Friedrich Schiller

AS YOU LIVE WITH CERTAINTY the goal is to remain ever aware and aligned with both your purposeful authenticity and the flow of your spiritual power frequency. This puts you in the best, most optimal place to receive messages and guidance from the universe. Your daily life is infused with this guidance and communication. You need only raise your awareness, have faith, and take the time to recognize and digest these messages. Seemingly mundane, everyday events and commonplace occurrences can carry great importance, meaning, and consequence when you awaken to their existence.

Developing an awareness of signs and important messages from the Spirit dimension provides you with a backstage pass to the workings of Source energy. Even if you've never before noticed such guidance, rest assured that this phenomenon applies to you. The universe speaks to every single one of us through myriad signs and messages throughout our lives. In the past, you may not have paid much attention to them because it was more convenient to write them off as coincidence, particularly if the message wasn't obvious. As you live with certainty, you'll increasingly notice nudges or jolts from Source energy.

What Are Signs, Symbols, Signals, and Synchronicities?
The entire universe is linked and interconnected through energy. Energy is the medium for guidance and messages intended to help

you in your endeavor to co-create your life through interplay with Source energy.

The universe communicates with us through signs, signals, symbols, and synchronicities that transcend words. These energetic impulses are a resource for us as we move through life in our physical forms. The key is to remain aware as guidance unfolds. These personal messages connect us to our transcendent selves, and are proof of our innate interconnectivity with all things throughout the universe. As you come to understand and accept Source energy's presence, and begin to recognize the ways in which it filters into your physical existence, you'll gradually become infused with heightened insight that helps define your individual purpose.

By living with certainty, you dial into your optimal vibrational frequency and invite signs and synchronicities that further enable you to work in sync with Source energy. As you recognize and follow the signs, you are in essence following your intuition.

Communication and guidance from Source energy will fill your life with vitality and assurance. These signs, signals, symbols, and synchronicities serve as guidance and also:

- Represent pure and powerful communication from the Spirit dimension
- Infuse you with faith and trust that Source energy loves you, is with you, and is confirming and affirming your existence
- Open doors for you, keeping you in alignment with Source energy and your inspired soul-view
- Provide specific lessons, answers, guidance, opportunities, and messages directly from Source energy about your life path and development
- Provide you with the universe's feedback, either affirming your approach or guiding you back on track
- Offer doubt and warnings regarding decisions and actions, sending you messages that may show you the way out of a negative circumstance
- Provide a reflection of how you've been living, and changes

that may be necessary in order to live in alignment with your inspired soul-view
- Help you to face challenges with faith and strength and to make inspired soul-view-aligned decisions and choices
- Bring a vital element to your life that causes you to engage with life and nature in an interconnected manner

It is important to note that we can become so focused on connecting the positive dots that we're taken aback when the dots connect in ways that we don't expect—but this, too, is guidance for which we should be grateful. Specific messages may be intended to provide you with warnings that there is energy building around a certain person or circumstance. You must remain aware as the pieces of the puzzle fall into place, while accepting that even the most energy-draining, negative encounters are also part of growing and learning.

The Tradition of Signs
Historically, signs and symbols have played a meaningful role in human life and spirituality. As recently as one hundred years ago, people found it more natural and comfortable to discuss the role that signs and synchronicities play in our lives. People embraced the concept of universal interconnectivity and understood that signs appeared for everyone. The interpretation of signs and symbols was comfortable and familiar, because people lived much closer to nature, and had a deeper sense of interconnectivity to their fellow humans and the life surrounding them. The most common signs involved nature, and in general, people felt a far more intrinsic connection toward the land.

A mere century later, huge advances in technology have significantly changed how we live. Individualism and isolation have become more the norm, yet some of the most successful people ever to have walked the Earth possessed a keen instinct about energy, and how it impacted their lives. They lived with a certainty that there was a higher guidance aligned with their purpose.

Experiencing Signs—How They Appear

So where do you look to find these signs and symbols? It's simple—Source energy provides you with this guidance as you move through your daily life. All you have to do is to remain aware. Oftentimes, the busyness that you drape over yourself—and, consequently, your soul—smothers any awareness of these signs. Or, you may not recognize messages until they're so obvious that they clobber you over the head. Even then, you may still be tempted to dismiss them as coincidence.

Start simple. Look at cloud formations, street signs, numbers, people, days, and dates. Anything that catches your eye and strikes you as noteworthy may be a message. Don't force anything. As the flow of your spiritual power frequency develops, signs and synchronicities will become more obvious.

Don't expect to hear words or voices—typically, signs don't appear this way, though there are exceptions. Most likely, you'll see or experience signs through an aspect of your daily life—through an interaction, event, visual cue, circumstance, or even déjà vu. Signs are metaphorical. The content of the sign itself may have meaning for you, or may catch your attention because of its repetition or "seriality." Paul Kammerer, an Austrian biologist (1881–1926), coined the term seriality for things that repeat themselves over time.[2] Numbers, letters, words, phrases, or symbols can repeatedly appear, even in our dreams.

Signs are dynamic, can appear singularly or as seriality, and may include any number of symbols, typically visual, including the following:

- **Conversation and Dialogue.** Signs may appear in your own conversations or in overheard conversations that echo deeply within you, providing a light-bulb moment, as if the conversation was intended specifically for you to overhear. There may be implications relative to your current circumstances.
- **Dreams.** Often, dreams convey messages ranging from circumstances to people to your health, and even serve as portents of the future.

Chapter 4: Signs, Signals, Symbols, and Synchronicities

- **Inanimate Objects.** Absolutely any article—a clock, crucifix, or flag—that is recurring, or appears synchronistically, can be a sign. An object may appear where you don't recall leaving it, triggering a meaning, thought, or idea. Take note when an object appears in a peculiar place.
- **Letters, Words, and Numbers.** You may hear or see the same word, letter, or number repeat on a billboard, in the newspaper, on a license plate, in an email, and on the radio all on the same day. Even lyrics and specific phrases may begin repeating for you.
- **Nature, Animals, and Insects.** Powerful and compelling signs can be delivered through our interaction with nature, including animals, weather, wind, clouds, gems, stones, and trees.
- **People.** Consider it a sign or guidance when you dream or think of the same person repeatedly.
- **Random Thoughts.** Thoughts that may initially seem forgettable or insignificant may leave behind or spark thought-provoking signs or messages.
- **Synchronous Events.** Seeming coincidences may be the universe communicating a message to you.
- **Unanticipated Assistance, Uncanny Luck, or Support at Just the Right Moment.** These events can be direct messages from the universe.

As you live with certainty, you'll learn to view everything that happens to you through the lens of awareness. When you take a wrong turn, get a wrong-number call, or miss your train, take note of what was going through your mind, and stay on the lookout for repetition. When the same signs appear repeatedly, there's something to it. The universe won't give up until it is sure that you've received the message.

Interpreting and Translating Abstract Messages

Once you see a sign or synchronicity, then what? How do you discern the meaning, opportunity, or lesson? Recognizing and understanding signs and symbolism requires conscious effort. You have to pay attention, listen, be present, and above all, trust your intuition and instinct. We all are hardwired with the ability to see and read signs. Think of it as our "uncommon sense."

Each synchronistic event is highly personal, and you are the only person who can truly translate and interpret how the meaning pertains to your own life. When a sign is real and intended for you, your instinct will tell you beyond the shadow of any doubt that you are experiencing guidance.

Current circumstances must always be taken into consideration when trying to decipher a message or sign. Consider the environment and circumstances in which the event occurred relative to what is going on in your heart, mind, and overall psyche at that moment. Signs can show you the relationship between an Earthly event and your inner mindset. Sometimes the message is meant to show you some aspect of yourself that you need to heal or fix. Or, it may simply be to direct you to your subconscious. Roll it around in your mind. All that matters is that you take note and interpret the meaning for yourself.

Signs will change as you do, and you must interpret them based on where you are in your life. A sign that catches your attention at one time may mean nothing at a later time. A very faint or subtle sign may take some time to decipher, while other messages may be obvious. Keep track of what's been said, or what has transpired as a result, because the meaning may not be apparent until some time later. If you cannot decipher the meaning of a sign or synchronous event, ask your subconscious mind what it means, and then meditate on the answer. Watch for the kinds of images and thoughts that cross your mind during your meditative state. What emotions come to the surface as you reflect upon a sign? Listen for the message using all of your senses, including physical sensations, thoughts that come to mind, and what your intuition tells you.

Abstract symbols, signs, and circumstances can and do carry powerful messages from the spirit realm to the physical realm. You may find it useful to keep a journal or record of the signs and symbols that have held significance for you during your life.

Coincidence or Synchronicity?

A coincidence is a remarkable occurrence of similar or corresponding events happening together at the same time by chance, apparently without reason. We've all experienced coincidences. Often, we try to explain away our intuition that we have just experienced a synchronistic event by saying, "I just got lucky" or "I was simply in the right place at the right time." We take note for a moment before shrugging off any possibility of deeper meaning. However, I reject the notion that all inexplicable occurrences always fall into the category of haphazard, meaningless coincidence.

It has been said that coincidence occurs roughly 20% of the time, but what about the other 80%? If a part of you suspects that there may be other forces at work on your behalf, you're absolutely right. Living with certainty necessitates the faith to accept that so-called "coincidences," particularly those that align with the Earthly unfolding of your inspired soul-view and purposeful authenticity, are communication from Source energy. You must open yourself to the greater implication behind compelling experiences that you intuit to be more than random coincidence. Trust that when you receive a sign or message seemingly out of the blue, or at the best possible time, the universe is speaking to you. When circumstances align perfectly, it's time to acknowledge and express gratitude for the universal hand of grace at work in the unfolding of your life.

Carl Gustav Jung (1875–1961), a Swiss psychologist and the founder of analytical psychology, developed the term synchronicity to describe the coincidental events linking mind and matter that cannot be explained through cause and effect. These mystical coincidences carry powerful messages from the universe.

Grace and synchronicity are one and the same—a loving aspect of the universe that encourages, assists, and collaborates with us on our journey. Synchronicity gives us a glimpse of how the universe works with us, hears us, and supports us in an effort to bring us into alignment with universal forces, and demonstrates that we are part of the universe's interconnected grand design.

Synchronicity is a simultaneous coming together of event, time, and place that appears to be spiritually arranged in order to provide us with needed, timely guidance. Synchronous events are highly improbable, seemingly random events that carry significant personal meaning and timing, and the chance that they would occur together randomly must be so small that it defies statistical probability. To the spiritually awakened, these occurrences happen or repeat too frequently to be disregarded as mere chance. They are openings afforded to us by the universe, and our only job is to be aware of the guidance, live with heightened intuition, and walk through the opening. Synchronicities can be immensely comforting because they grab and focus your awareness on the supreme, universal harmonizing energy operating in your life.

Universal Interconnectivity

The notion of universal interconnectivity and Oneness is intrinsic to the concept of synchronicity. A deep interconnection and meaning lies behind signs, symbols, signals, and synchronicities. Thanks to the complex web of energy to which we are all interconnected, there are no random events; even seemingly distinct and unrelated events are connected. As you live with certainty, you begin perceiving your life and surroundings as deliberate, and accept that every person who crosses your path through any sort of interaction or conversation is there for a reason. They have some purpose, something to teach you within the overall universal web relative to your life. When seemingly random and disconnected outer events connect with your emotions, dreams, activities, and passions, it leaves no room for doubt that you're connected to everything and everyone in the universe.

Frequency 19

Many years ago, I discovered that when a significant event transpired

Chapter 4: Signs, Signals, Symbols, and Synchronicities

personally or professionally—or when I was repeatedly blessed with the very things I so desired—somehow, some way the number 19 was nearly always present. Over time I came to realize that my highest vibrating energy—that of love and compassion—somehow aligns with number 19. With each appearance, I physically feel my heart open as I experience a vibrational alignment with Source energy. I know with certainty that together we are co-creating the life the universe always intended for me to live—the life that my soul entered into Earthly physicality to experience.

Over the years, I've had periods of time when the 19s were nowhere to be found. The lack of high-energy resonance in my body was palpable. I believe the number 19 repeats at times when I am clearly aligned with the flow of my spiritual power frequency. The number of 19s that I see has been so inexplicable that I came to realize that they were being shown to me as a result of my feelings, thoughts, beliefs, and how I was living my life. They have always been a sign that lets me know when my energy is vibrating at a high frequency. I experience all manner of other signs, signals, symbols, and synchronicities as well, but the number 19 remains consistent. When my energy aligns with the flow of my spiritual power frequency, it's like tuning my internal energy dial to the frequency that allows me to co-create my life—I call it "Frequency 19." When I am in the flow of this powerful alignment, good things occur at a fast pace, and signs and synchronicities reveal themselves at every turn. (Not insignificantly, Paul Kammerer's book referenced earlier was published in 1919.)

By no means did I set out to find a number to which I was incredibly sensitive, but over time I recognized that 19 was revealing itself to me. Through that revealing, my world opened up for me a direct connection to the spiritual plane that has guided me to the greatest joys of my life. Frequency 19 enables me—mind, body, and spirit—to feel inspired and deeply hopeful, while reinforcing that we live in a mysterious, interconnected universe.

The number 19 has appeared for me in any number of ways that are just part of my daily life. When a 19 appears, I have conditioned myself to take note of what I was thinking at that moment. The key is not that I remain on the lookout for any old 19 (we are all surrounded by advertisers who go to great lengths to make sure we don't miss their numbers and signs), but for me they appear with seriality while invoking powerful instinct. Here are some examples of the ways the number 19 has appeared in my life.

- My daughter was born in a Minneapolis hospital in Room 19—and, no, I did not request that room. As a matter of fact, I didn't notice the room number posted on the wall behind my bed until five years after her birth, while watching the birth video.
- While driving on the freeway, School Bus 19 merged in front of me immediately causing me to reduce my speed from 65 mph to 35 mph. In so doing, Bus 19 saved me from driving directly behind an old pickup truck whose rear tailgate blew off and would have landed on my car. Thankfully, Bus 19 created significant space between our vehicles.
- My father died on July 19.
- My office phone port number in the workroom was 19.
- All mail forwarded to my home office from a downtown office has a 19 hand-written on the envelope, without a who or why.
- On a trip to Aspen, the first restaurant we saw as we rounded the corner from our hotel was named 19.
- I asked someone the time and they respond in military time, 19:19.
- My first cheerleading tryout number was 19.
- A lunch bill with a friend was split and we each received a credit card receipt for $19.19.
- Fire Engine 19 pulls up next to me at a stoplight.
- My plane arrived at gate 19 after I was seated in row 19.
- I arrive late to the airport only to be told that the flight moved to gate 19.

The appearance of the number 19 in my life has heightened my awareness in general, kept me aligned with flow, and provided me with guidance, assurance, and support at just the right time. I am so grateful for this aspect of grace in my life.

Identifying Your Personal Signs

As you raise your awareness, you will become more attuned to your intuition and how your personal energy is vibrating. Signs and synchronicities will reveal themselves repeatedly and consistently to you in a way that will be instinctively obvious. When you find an affirmative pattern, sign, or number, there will be no mistaking it. You'll see the repetition; you'll feel your groove.

Here's a wonderful example. We can assume that NASCAR racing great Darrell Waltrip has a positive energetic alignment with number 17. On February 17, he won the Daytona 500 on his 17th attempt while driving car No.17 that was pitted in Stall 17 when his daughter was 17 months old. He co-creates the life the universe always intended for him to live when his energy is vibrating optimally as Frequency 17.[3]

Sign Skeptics

Why be skeptical? What harm can come from living with awareness and in alignment with your instinct and intuition while allowing signs, signals, symbols, and synchronicities to guide your soul-view–aligned action? While skeptics try to disregard synchronicities as nothing more than random events or coincidence, to live with certainty is to believe in, and exist on, a higher plane. You can either choose to find the significance of signs, or you can choose to write them off as mere coincidence. If you choose the latter, you deny yourself the opportunity to receive guidance from the intelligence of the universe, and to co-create your life in concert with Source energy. Instead, why not consider the deeper meaning and personal possibilities?

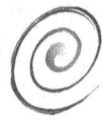

CHAPTER 5

Static

*"Don't overlook small and seemingly insignificant negative actions.
The smallest of sparks can burn down a mountain."*
—Tibetan saying

MOST OF US THINK of static as the noise produced in a radio or television receiver by atmospheric or other electrical disturbances that prevent electricity from flowing as current. Within the context of Living with Certainty, static refers to the dense, negative, self-limiting white noise and distortion within your being that lowers your personal vibrational frequency.

Spiritually, static is weakening and draining. As static weakens your spirit, it also disturbs the flow of your spiritual power frequency, which is an extremely delicate state. As you engage in thoughts, intentions, activities, and behaviors that are not giving, loving, and compassionate, you create energy blockages and resistance that lower your vibrational frequency and weaken your alignment with Source energy, affecting your purposeful authenticity. As static blocks the exchange of positive energy, it counteracts your ability to co-create the life the universe always intended for you to live.

Junk energy—negative emotion, unproductive thought, unhealthy ego, distorted perceptions—adds toxicity to your entire system; not just mentally, but also physically and spiritually. This jams and scrambles your personal vibrational frequency. You may routinely find yourself facing blockages and impasses due to unintentional negative mindsets created by your ego-personality. Whatever the specifics, as you experience negative, unproductive emotions, you produce an overall negative energy that's inherently dense and low-vibrating. This negative energy may even set into motion karma that is not in alignment with anything that you want.

Static is akin to a piano that's out of tune—regardless of the skill and effort put forth to play the notes, the instrument is off-key, and the song will not be sweet. Similarly, if you choose to engage in such things as unethical behavior or addictions, your instrument—in this case your mind, body, and spirit—will not be in tune. The irony is that the presence of static is a clear indicator that through your own efforts, you're blocking yourself from receiving what you want. Static impedes forward movement. You can't expect to align with the universe's most pure energy when you're in a negative state. Instead, you'll place yourself in the perfect place for attracting even more negativity—precisely what you don't want.

How Does Static Feel?

Remember what it's like to receive a shock from static electricity, such as a small shock from touching a doorknob? What you experience is a burst of electricity, rather than a steady, easy flow. This is similar to the effect of dense, negative energy that can be created through actions, thoughts, or beliefs. It blocks the flow of loving, high-frequency energy, and allows a shock of negativity to become absorbed into your being. Immediately, you feel bad. This energy blockage leaves you feeling spiritually anemic, weak, heavy, and muddled. You move through the days without the clarity, love, and gratitude that sustain your connection to your spiritual power frequency and Source energy.

These same negative emotions also serve as your internal instruction system, alerting you to the fact that you're out of alignment with your purposeful authenticity. Something is wrong. These feelings provide a warning that you're engaged in something that's not right for you. You may experience a sense of isolation or loneliness as these negative emotions weaken your alignment with your positive energy flow and your subconscious sense of universal interconnectivity. When you find yourself in this state, you must consciously and immediately transform how you are thinking and relating to your world.

Once you know what it feels like to be aligned with the flow of your spiritual power frequency and to vibrate fine, high-frequency energy, you will easily sense when your energy becomes dense and low-vibrating. During those inevitable times when life isn't going smoothly and you're feeling negative, defeated, or just generally blue, take stock of your feelings. Maybe your thoughts and words have become negative and pessimistic, or you are obsessively running the same negative loop about the past over and over in your mind. Feeling like a victim trapped by circumstance, remaining in negative relationships, or feeling envious of what others have are all thoughts and feelings that create static, and must be eliminated. You may be surprised to understand the full spectrum of Earthly actions, beliefs, feelings, and thoughts that induce static and block you from experiencing your inspired soul-view and deep-soul joy (see the *Living with Certainty Discovery Guide* for a full list). Life-long conditioning can be so powerful that you move through life with blinders on. Many people tend to collect the negative experiences of their lives, giving weight and power to old baggage, thus tipping the balance of their overall mental health toward the dark side.

Removing Static

You must learn to eliminate the noise and toxicity of static from your vibrational frequency. As you do this and it becomes your natural approach to life, you'll find that doubt, pessimism, disbelief, and other toxic feelings will become less intense and habitual.

You can't always control external circumstances, but you can control their effect on you. You've likely experienced times when you're in a great mood, only to have someone spoil it with his or her depressing problems or pessimistic attitude. How do you cope when you feel you could live with certainty if only the people in your life—family, co-workers, even strangers—would stop bringing you down?

First, it's important to practice Living with Certainty in its totality and with great commitment. Many of the 65 Living with Certainty

Energy Enablers you'll learn about in Part 3 specifically teach you how to cope with these situations. Next, the easiest and most powerful way to begin is to give thanks and gratitude for the presence of these characters in your life. At some point, they must have possessed sterling qualities that attracted you. These people may not be receiving much positive reinforcement in their daily lives, so heap praise on them for whatever good qualities they do have, and attempt to serve as an uplifting example to them. In addition, be grateful for the lessons you have learned from them about how not to live.

As for truly negative people, limit your exposure to them as much as you can. Clearly, this is difficult when the person is a co-worker or family member. When inevitable conflict arises, avoid arguments, debate, antagonism, and extensive conversations that only serve to lengthen your exposure to them. Don't judge them, don't spend time stewing over them or hating them—just interact to the extent that you have to and then let the interaction go. You can't afford to let their negativity lower your own vibrational frequency and destroy your ability to co-create your life.

Your awareness of how static feels, and your ability to immediately shift your focus to something more positive, will allow you to strengthen your spiritual power frequency. As your awareness develops and static dissipates, you will immediately notice a difference in how you feel. Energy vibrations immediately lighten and rise to higher frequency levels as your exchange with Source energy once again to flow freely.

Where to begin? When you are calm, you have the potential to be more objective. Daily meditation can work wonders in bringing calm and peace to your life, enabling you objectively to assess your circumstances. Two effective methods that can help you to find your calm center when events around you become tense or chaotic are to take on the perspective of an observer, not an active participant; and to use your Sacred Sevens.

Sacred Sevens is a deep-breathing technique targeted at slowing the heart rate, decreasing the release of adrenaline, increasing oxygen, lowering blood pressure, and increasing the release of natural, feel-good chemicals called endorphins. The technique is simple: breathe deeply from your abdomen, inhale slowly and gently for seven seconds, hold the breath for seven seconds, and then exhale slowly for seven seconds with conscious intent to release and breathe out all negativity.

You can always practice your Sacred Sevens, regardless of your physical location. If you feel an anxiety attack coming on, or feel yourself becoming upset about something, your Sacred Sevens can help calm you by allowing you to reconnect with your soul-center through conscious thought and breath. Use this technique when you feel stressed, anxious, or overwhelmed. You'll become more aware of the here and now moment, and regain a clearer sense of priorities.

Leaving Your Frequency ... Temporarily

Why do we move in and out of alignment with the flow of our spiritual power frequency? One day, things are happening at a fast and dynamic pace just as we want—and the next day everything falls apart. For starters, we're human and susceptible to life's unavoidable ups and downs. Our minds wander constantly, imagining countless problems and outcomes. We may have put forth great effort to live with certainty, only to find that for three weeks, two months, or longer we've become disconnected from the flow of our spiritual power frequency. Why? How did this happen, and how do we restore this vital connection?

When you sense that your alignment with the flow of your spiritual power frequency has weakened, spend a few minutes in reflection and introspection regarding your recent intentions and actions. Try to understand the nature of the misalignment between your life and your purposeful authenticity. Meditate, be still, and pray. Become keenly aware of signs, signals, symbols, and synchronicities. No signs? No synchronous events? Just a dull, down feeling? You may very well be headed down the wrong path, not living in alignment with your inspired soul-view. If you feel that you're neither aligned with your spiritual power frequency, nor receiving guidance or communication from the universe, you may have more internal work to do. It may be time to regroup, slow down, and meditate. Be honest with yourself about any recent actions, thoughts, intentions, and choices that could be dulling your energy and creating static.

Static will inevitably creep into your vibrational frequency from time to time—your ego will see to it. Remain proactive and be selective in your focus. As life happens to your body and mind, it remains your choice whether or not you let it negatively impact your spirit.

Relax into Your Faith as You Live with Certainty

You may feel that you are doing everything with all of your might, and yet still nothing is working. This could be because you're pushing too hard. Ironically, by desperately attempting to force your power to co-create, you can weaken your abilities.

Once you accept that you are intrinsically connected to Source energy, there's no need to struggle or force anything. Attempting to get rough with the universe only adds static to your vibrational frequency and gets you nowhere. Engaging in any control-based activity actually creates frustration and static because you're not operating from a place of absolute faith. In the back of your mind is a pocket of disbelief or doubt.

However, once you align with your inspired soul-view, you'll believe that the life the universe always intended for you to live is already yours. As you move through your day engaged in purposeful activities and continually expressing gratitude, you vibrate energy that makes yourself and others feel good. Everything else will take care of itself if you just allow it.

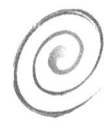

PART II

Discovering the Life the Universe Always Intended for You to Live

*"Man is his own star; and the soul that can
Render an honest and perfect man,
Commands all light, all influence, all fate;
Nothing to him falls early or too late."*
—Ralph Waldo Emerson

Your time in Earthly physicality is not separate from the ethereal plane of existence from which your soul emerged. You simultaneously straddle both realms through the energy of your soul. Everything essential to enlightenment and transformation exists within you at this very moment. Here, now, today, you can begin to co-create the life the universe always intended for you to live. This is a life of deep-soul joy, characterized by the fullest expression of your purposeful authenticity. It is your most authentic, fulfilling, inspired, and abundant life made manifest, embracing every aspect of your unseen self—your spirit, passions, creativity, instincts, dreams, and revelations.

When you live the life the universe always intended for you to live, every life experience contributes to your personal development and enlightenment. This is your soul's intended Earthly path—full of pain and ecstasy, disappointment and joy. Begin now to take responsibility for your inner, spiritual life as outlined in the following chapters. You have the power.

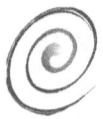

CHAPTER 6

Your Inspired Soul-View

"All suffering comes from believing ourselves to be what we are not. We think we are a body and personality that is born to die, but our true identity is unborn and so never dying. We are the Mind of the universe. The separate ego-self is a phantom with no essential reality."
—Timothy Freke

AT THE MERE MENTION of the word "spirituality" some people start to squirm. They don't know how to define it, they're not comfortable discussing it, and they may be fearful of what is actually *out there*.

The word spirituality refers to the human spirit or soul. Your spirit is simply the higher consciousness aspect of yourself that inhabits your body. Spirituality encompasses the awareness and appreciation of the fact that you are connected to Source energy. It allows you to view the world with deeper meaning, significance, harmony, and universal interconnectivity. It fuels the journey of your personal quest for truth—about yourself, the workings of the universe, and your reason for being.

It is a fundamental aspect of our nature to be curious about how the universe works and where we fit in. Spirituality encompasses lucid, coherent, and intelligent thought. The time we spend in Earthly physicality is intended for spiritual evolution with the goal of diminishing the stronghold of our ego and bringing us to our inspired soul-view. As we evolve spiritually, we are able to receive and experience deep-soul joy, the overarching purpose of our Earthly lives. The aim is to become indisputably aware, authentic, and bold enough to pursue your dreams and deepest joy. This can only be achieved through a spiritual life. This isn't to say that atheists can't have a good Earthly life—certainly, they can; but they are not living with the depth of purposeful authenticity and deep-soul joy that the spiritually enlightened enjoy.

We Are First and Foremost Spirit

Humans are first and foremost Spirit, or soul, experiencing the physical dimensions of Earth—not the other way around. Your inspired soul-view is an extension of Source energy. Dr. Susan Gregg describes the human spirit in her book, *The Complete Idiot's Guide to Spiritual Healing.* She says, "Your spirit is limitless; it is without bounds; it is immortal; and it is infinite. Anything that stops you from experiencing yourself as that spirit limits your joyous experience of life."[4]

The authentic You can only be found within the essence of your soul; you are not just a brain, body, ego, or mind. Your physical body and your ego-personality are merely what the world sees. But this pure energy of the soul that dwells within you is just as real as your Earthly physical body. The energy of your soul enters into Earthly physicality in order to develop, grow, learn, and heal.

Your soul is the transcendent, deep, limitless aspect of your being; it is the essence and fundamental nature of who you really are. Your soul has been the contiguous essence of yourself that's been with you throughout your life's journey. Your soul does not know time, limits, or constraints—only the pure energy of love, service, and compassion. Only when you tap into that essence and become fully aware of its inspiration will you begin to know yourself.

Up until now you may have neglected exploring this aspect of your being, despite the fact that you sense its presence or have had hints of awareness that another energy plane exists. These fleeting moments of awareness may not yet have proven intense enough for you to abandon your familiar conditioning. It may have felt safer to embrace only the Earthly dimension that you can see and directly experience. If you're not occasionally glimpsing the presence of another dimension in your life, you're not living with awareness—the signs are there for you, just as they are for each of us.

No Religion Required

Being spiritual does not mean practicing a specific religion. Many people live highly spiritual lives connected to Source energy without practicing any formal religion. At the same time, many self-proclaimed religious people are not at all spiritually enlightened. Choose the spiritual path that's right for you. Find a practice that brings you equilibrium and real peace. Spirituality knows no boundaries, no ethnicities, no social economics.

Source Energy

Through your inspired soul-view, you are connected to Source energy. True fulfillment comes only when your essence welcomes and incorporates Source energy into your daily existence. Only you and all-knowing Source energy have any real power over your spiritual life. When you live according to your inspired soul-view, you are moved and motivated by the command, strength, and force of Source energy as it works in tandem with you to bring into Earthly form the life the universe always intended for you to live.

When Source energy is co-guiding your efforts, no dream is too big or too impossible. The specific purpose of your life is not a mystery: somehow, some way, you are intrinsically interconnected with the Universe's greater plan to spread love and joy.

The Greatest Gift You Can Give Yourself

The most significant revelation, and the single greatest honor and opportunity of your lifetime, is to discover and live in alignment with your inspired soul-view. Much of the torment and misery that is present in the world stems from our inability to live from our souls.

At one time or another, you may have experienced emptiness and longing that typically results from one of two causes. First, your inspired soul-view may be attempting to raise your awareness of its existence. Consider this feeling of unrest to be a call to action—your call to awaken the inspired soul-view that is yearning to express itself. At your core, you know who you are, why you are here, and whether or not you are living in alignment with your purposeful authenticity. If you're not, your soul will let you know. Second, some people believe that these feelings can appear when you are in a spiritual transition to the next level of your Earthly existence. Your soul may be adjusting and preparing for the next phase of your life.

When we are not living in alignment with our Earthly purpose, our souls feel confined and restricted. Think for a moment how you have attempted to fill this emptiness in the past—by jumping from one hollow relationship to another, overindulging in alcohol and parties, shopping or buying new toys, having yet another child. These are all outside solutions. The only real, lasting solution is to create from the inside a life that is a pure expression of your purposeful authenticity.

You were born with the ability, tools, and hardwiring to bring forth your inspired soul-view. Your life's work is simply to awaken and align with it. You must learn to let go of your ego, surrender to your internal instruction system, and take aligned action along the path of the life the universe always intended for you to live. You must live every day by building a more total alignment between your thoughts, actions, beliefs, emotions, and inspired soul-view.

Your Inspired Soul-View

Your inspired soul-view, the formless You, dwells in your spirit-core—that place in your physical being that vibrates with spiritual energy. The core of this energy resides in your chest, solar plexus, and heart. Consider your soul to be a loving, peaceful, and safe place in your heart, not in your mind, brain, or thoughts. It is helpful to think of your soul as living in your heart, because it reprograms you to stop listening to only the thoughts in your head. Just as you don't need to think about it to know that your heart is beating, you need only stop, become aware, and feel what your inspired soul-view is conveying.

I refer to the soul as your inspired soul-view because your soul is inspiration, infusing your being with authenticity, purpose, and insight as to how to live life in expression of your intended Earthly purpose. Many successful people describe having a difficult-to-articulate, yet firm sense from their earliest years that they were destined for greatness. This is their inspired soul-view coming through. Discovering and becoming aware of these messages means that you are paying attention to your intuition.

Your soul knows what you really require to experience deep-soul joy. Your ego thinks it knows, but in reality your ego has absolutely no connection to, or knowledge of, your inspired soul-view. Your inspired soul-view has nothing to do with how much you own or how much money you make. It is not your ego, possessions, profession, or education; nor is it the pursuit of frivolous pleasures or desires. It is, instead, all things based in love, service, and compassion.

Your inspired soul-view is unique to your own needs for growth, healing, and development. However, in broad terms, all souls share certain characteristics. Your inspired soul-view:

- Is your access to Source energy's complete knowledge about your Earthly purpose
- Is your internal core of authenticity, wisdom, and clarity
- Provides what is best for you at all times
- Is the infinite, perfect, invisible you
- Has no boundaries
- Demands complete awareness and living in the here and now
- Requires that you embrace openness and trust your intuition
- Is the authentic you—regardless of your health, thoughts, or energy level
- Is always there—the essence behind your Earthly physicality
- Contains no judgment, no past, no regrets

What are the ramifications of living in alignment with your inspired soul-view? You are optimally vibrating energy as you create a life that is an expression of your purposeful authenticity. Your energy comes as close as possible to the vibrational frequency of Source energy. It is a daily joy to co-create your heart's desire when you work in sync with the same purpose as Source energy.

Your Intention to Discover Your Inspired Soul-View

As you begin the journey to discover your inspired soul-view, find a spot where you're surrounded by natural splendor. Sit in stillness outside on a crystal clear night contemplating the stars or on a beach gazing out at the ocean. If you're fortunate to live near a majestic mountain range, take in the snow-capped, spellbinding views. You'll unmistakably feel the universe's powerful natural energy and sense your interconnectedness with all of existence.

The process of discovering your inspired soul-view begins with the firm intention to do so, coupled with the essential first steps of developing awareness, stillness, and surrender. Inner peace laced with intention is the path to discovering your inspired soul-view. You must rise above the notion that you're nothing more than Earthly physicality bound by Earthly limitations. The intent to live the rest of your life in awareness of your connection to Source energy is the beginning of the discovery process. Once you understand that you're intrinsically a part of Source energy, and make the decision to discover and express the unique gifts that you were put into Earthly physicality to share with the world, you're on your way.

We Are More Than Our Five Senses

Discovering your inspired soul-view is a journey that requires introspection and a commitment to develop your awareness beyond your five senses. The journey to your inspired soul-view requires attentiveness and an ability to tune out any static. This is a place of Divine connection, intuition, contentment, joy, and hunch. This place is you. You are already there. You cannot fail because Source energy is already with you—and always has been.

Your inspired soul-view has been communicating with you for your entire life, though you may not have been aware of its messages. Your soul is not concerned with communicating with you in terms that are easily understandable. It doesn't use words of language. It can be a feeling, hunch, smell, or sensation, but you must do the deciphering. As we saw in Chapter 4, physical and emotional signs, signals, symbols, and synchronicities provide affirmation that you are living in alignment with your inspired soul-view. Your inspired soul-view represents the enlightened you, but prepare yourself for the fact that you may not be who you thought you were.

Profound Connection

Your inspired soul-view creates a spectrum of states ranging from deep and intense, to subtle and faint. You must learn to quiet your mind if you are to discover and understand these subtle messages. As you connect with this depth of self-knowledge, it vibrates with you more profoundly than a typical thought ever could. At times the experience of your inspired soul-view is pure elation or deep-soul joy, causing you to tingle from head to toe with the experience of this alignment. You feel your connection to the Source in a very dynamic way—as if the pure energy love coursing through your essence is being transmitted back and forth between two ends of a lightning bolt.

Receive and Trust

It requires a leap of faith to follow your inspired soul-view. The more you notice these messages, the more frequently they'll appear. Don't judge your soul-view, or the associated yearnings to do certain things. Don't think, *This doesn't make any sense*, or *This will never work*. Go with your gut, and don't let anyone talk you out of what your gut is telling you. Have faith in this information without questioning it. There is no risk when you're creating more of what is good in the world—love, joy, tenderness, compassion, and sharing.

Negative Emotions

Your inspired soul-view uses positive emotion to communicate what you need to do in order to live the life the universe always intended for you to live. Right action feels aligned with a greater good. Negative feelings and emotions are signals and warnings that you are not aligned with your inspired soul-view. Keep in mind that when you have thoughts that are distinctly not soul-thoughts—those lacking in love, compassion, or good intentions—you have added static into your spiritual power frequency, and darkness is diminishing your connection. Your feelings will always let you know this.

Why You Must Live in Alignment with Your Inspired Soul-View

Why should we actively seek to access our inspired soul-view? Because it is a gift to experience this level of consciousness. This process of authentic self-soul discovery will lead to a higher state of consciousness. Once you live in alignment with your inspired soul-view, your life will begin to transform in ways that seem practically miraculous. This level of consciousness traverses Source energy and provides the joy, wisdom, and answers that you otherwise could not receive. Once achieved, you can begin to expand yourself and your life beyond the self-imposed, conditioned boundaries that you've lived with to date. For example:

- Your capacity to access deep-soul joy will be infinitely multiplied.
- You'll tap into the flow of your spiritual power frequency and feel a profound gratitude and reverence for the gift of life.
- Divine love and guidance will dwell within you.
- You'll gain peace knowing that your soul is part of the overarching mystical universe, and will live on after your Earthly body turns to dust.
- You can relax in the knowledge that your time on Earth is about finding your essence, not about acquiring things.
- You understand that you've made your life on Earth more difficult than it was ever intended to be by allowing your ego to drive your thoughts and actions.
- Your priorities, opinions, beliefs, and values will be transformed.
- You will welcome the flow of Source energy directly into your life, easily receiving messages, guidance, and signs that light your way.

How It Feels to Live in Alignment with Your Inspired Soul-View

You'll know that you've peeled back the layers to reveal your inspired soul-view when your sense of purposeful authenticity is palpable, keeping you centered in the knowledge that you are an eternal part of the universe. Very naturally, and without effort, you will feel joyous, vital, and energized. You will believe in your own limitless potential in a way you never thought possible. What does it feel like to live this way, and how will you know when you experience it? You may experience some or all of the following:

- A feeling of purposeful authenticity, and a sense that you have found a higher calling to serve your soul while serving others
- A sense of faith, and an absolute knowing that you are on track and everything will be okay
- A sense of fullness, as if you have found an essential piece of yourself that you have long known was missing
- Feelings of joy and energized fulfillment, and a sense of creativity and enthusiasm
- A sense of abundant and unlimited possibility
- A lightness of being—the sensation of no longer being confined to your body; feelings of buoyancy; pulsing, tingling emotional energy vibrations; intense emotions of love and hope
- A heightened awareness of all that is happening both within and around you; you are alert and engaged
- A sublime sense of love and compassion for yourself and every aspect of your life
- A sense that you have experienced a glimpse of another realm that has forever and immensely expanded your perspective
- A desire to share and serve

Above all, you feel with complete certainty and faith that you are loved, that you are not alone, that you are a powerful co-creator, and that you are a part of the Highest energy in the universe. All of this will come naturally and effortlessly once you live in alignment with your inspired soul-view.

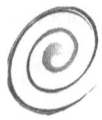

CHAPTER 7

Awareness

*"Let us not look back in anger or forward in fear,
but around in awareness."*
—James Thurber

YOUR DECISION TO FOLLOW a spiritual path and your commitment to live with certainty necessitates a practical, natural step-by-step process intended to help you awaken to your soul-based, authentic nature. Developing awareness is the essential first step to becoming both an astute observer and an active co-creator of your life. You can accomplish this by taking an objective perspective about what may be happening at any given moment, always aware of and assessing how you feel both emotionally and physically, and then taking soul-view-aligned action. From this high perch of awareness, you have a bird's-eye view to survey, examine, and co-create your life.

Learning to live from a state of deliberate, focused awareness is a requirement for living your most authentic life. It's a crucial component of keeping the sabotaging qualities of your ego-personality from emerging. Awareness allows you to notice, hear, learn from, and savor the here and now moments that create your experience and your life. Through both inward/internal and outward/external awareness you learn who you really are at the soul level. You'll no longer take anything for granted, and you will awaken to the beauty and experience of your Earthly life.

While you may not have developed or used it, awareness is an innate capability that you already possess. Approaching your life with awareness serves three primary purposes, each essential to living with certainty:

- Awareness creates a clear, static-free space where you will connect with and experience your inspired soul-view
- Awareness teaches you to live in the here and now, and to take perpetual measure of your surroundings
- Awareness teaches you to live your life with attentiveness to the nonverbal guides that serve you through your internal instruction system

What to Expect

As you awaken your awareness, you tap into the personal, clear space from which you can communicate and align with Source energy. This is where you'll begin to develop a profound sense of the authentic you and your inspired soul-view. As your awareness develops, the profound meaning and benefits of simply *being* will become clear to you. When you live from a state of perpetual awareness, you transform yourself and can expect to become more of the following:

- Accepting
- Authentic
- Connected
- Perceptive
- Free from the dense energy and the complexity of Earthly physicality
- Focused
- Observant
- Responsive
- Still
- Tolerant

Here and Now

Living a life of reverence and inspiration in alignment with your inspired soul-view requires that you remain completely attuned to how you feel here and now—not tomorrow or yesterday. Think of the moments of your life as dots, and your awareness as the line that connects them. If you allow your awareness line to dim, you'll miss the very moments in the present that reveal a whole world of possibilities. Living in the now is not a new concept. This core principle of Buddhism emphasizes that every aspect of life is fleeting and transitory. You have only the present moment you are experiencing; there is nothing else. Your only real power resides in the here and now, in being present and engaged in your thoughts and behavior, not in the past or the future. It's vital that you live in the present moment and experience what is happening within and around you now, allowing your heightened awareness to pull you away from the controlling grip of ego. Here, you will see the sights, hear the sounds, smell the aromas, taste the flavors, feel your emotions, and follow your instinct.

Be honest—how much time do you spend each day hoping and planning for the future, or stewing over the past? When you're obsessing over your thoughts and internal states, you're not living with an aligned awareness. Instead, you're allowing the real moments of life to pass you by. When you're preoccupied and filled to capacity with Earthly density, you deny yourself the opportunity to experience joy or learning.

The key to heightening your awareness is developing the ability to truly engage with your experience—to feel and learn from the message—without judging it. To do so, it's imperative that you allow your feelings to flow through you without becoming attached to them. Earthly ego-drivers that trigger a torrent of emotions are merely convenient cover-ups that allow the truth of the moment to slide away. It's far easier to be unthinking, unaware, and unconnected, and to allow your undisciplined ego to fill your Earthly self with soulless efforts. In fact, many people are so uncomfortable dealing with their present feelings that they'd rather think about memories, inconsequential topics, or even future events instead.

With awareness, you create room to remain open, soft, and malleable. Particularly during your most trying times, attempt to remain open to your emotions without blocking or ignoring them. This is when solutions, intuition, signs, and guidance appear.

It can be hard to stay in the moment. The best approach is simply to develop awareness as a habit. When you find yourself deep in thoughts of the past or future, simply tell yourself—either silently or aloud—*I am aware*. You'll know that you've made progress in developing awareness when you're able to catch yourself becoming swept away by emotion-inducing thoughts, and yet bring yourself back to awareness before you've weakened your alignment with the flow of your spiritual power frequency.

Awareness requires you to stop focusing on how things could be different, and focus instead on the present moment at hand. Think in terms of how Source energy would see the present moment you have been trying to avoid or change. Begin enjoying life's seconds, minutes, and hours, instead of focusing on the past or future.

Energy

Living in tune with energy—the universe's means of communicating with you—requires that you create a still space of gratitude and awareness from whence you can both receive and process messages. The greater your ability to tune in, the more powerful your alignment with the flow of your spiritual power frequency. You must be awake to everything happening around you, regardless of how seemingly insignificant. This is necessary if you are to live in alignment with the flow of your spiritual power frequency, and be receptive to the guidance provided to you through your internal instruction system.

Think of it as a radio or television in your home. No matter how many station signals are being transmitted, you won't receive any of them unless the television or radio is tuned in. The ability to cut off knee-jerk, judgmental thoughts and reactions is precisely what allows you to see the signs and hear the messages the universe is sending you. It's through your awareness that you'll notice peculiarities, random thoughts, patterns, unusual circumstances, signs, and synchronous events. These phenomena will illuminate your advancement and evolution while confirming for you that you are on the right life track and aligned with your inspired soul-view.

Your faith in the universe's ongoing presence in your life through its continuous communication and guidance must be accompanied by vigilant awareness. With awareness, epiphanies and revelations—even about significant life choices—come easier and with a certainty that cannot be experienced when the ego-personality is in charge. This reinforces your trust and faith in the fact that you are not alone.

Awakening to Awareness

Your intention to develop your awareness is an important beginning, but the process of working to raise your awareness is never-ending. Peeling back enough layers to experience awareness is an intense process that requires you to stop skimming the surface of your life, and to begin looking more deeply at people, events, and emotions. In this way, you'll begin to uncover the spiritual dimension and deeper meaning of how experiences or situations are related to your journey and to the universe.

As you begin the awareness journey, you must learn to be still. Within stillness and awareness is Spirit. Every moment you can spend sitting in stillness and in silent awareness is a gift. Focus your entire being in the here and now. Listen, sense, intuit, see, taste, feel, experience. Allow the still, empty space that you create to be an openness that envelops you at all times. Regardless of how chaotic your circumstances are you can always walk away, even if that requires walking into a closet for a moment just to be. Focus on your breath and realign with your soul-center. Practice your Sacred Sevens and allow your breath to restore your balance and your sense of universal interconnectivity with all of life.

It takes tremendous mindfulness and practice to develop awareness. In the beginning you have to catch yourself not being aware. Over time, this will come more naturally. We're all capable of heightening our awareness, just as we're all capable of becoming who we really are. The trick is not to allow yourself to lose your center as you move through your day. Though older, more mature adults generally seem to have a greater natural ability to live in the moment, absolutely anyone at any age at any time can develop their awareness.

Chapter 7: Awareness

After you've practiced catching yourself not being aware, it's time to practice applying yourself to life's select moments—the true riches in your life. A simple moment can become an experience of true awakening and make it easier to notice subsequent revelatory moments. If the concept of awareness is new to you, start small and easy. Get a table at a sidewalk café and sit and observe as the world goes by. Take in your surroundings. Awareness enhances the Earthly experience for all of us. Enjoy the way your wine smells, the taste of just-picked raspberries, fresh basil, or crisp cherry tomatoes. Savor the sweet smell of your child's or partner's skin, or a new rose bud. Delight in a cloud formation, a deer nibbling grass on the side of the road, the pink and purple sunset, or the sound of your children's endless chatter and giggles. Notice how blue the sky is, or the stage of the moon. Watch the red robins in your backyard. Read with your children and watch how they process a word for the first time.

The key to developing your awareness lies in your ability to recognize and respect the spirit that resides in all living things, as well as the energy that comprises all matter. The extent to which you allow your spiritual essence to engage and direct your Earthly existence will define your awareness level.

Through heightened awareness, you'll gain a sense of your essence that may be quite different from how you have previously perceived yourself. This moment—right here, right now—is intended for the further development of your purposeful authenticity—and nothing else.

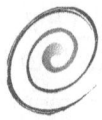

CHAPTER 8

Universal Interconnectivity

*"Within man is the soul of the whole; the wise silence;
the universal beauty, to which every part and particle
is equally related; the eternal one."*
—Ralph Waldo Emerson

AT THIS VERY MOMENT, every other part of the universe is interacting with your existence. Your life and the energy you vibrate intersects, crisscrosses, traverses, and overlaps with the lives and the energy of all of your fellow humans. Somehow, by some means, every aspect of our Earthly lives has been orchestrated in coordination with every other aspect of existence. Everything is inextricably linked. Consider the repercussions of this: What you may consider to be an inconsequential choice made during the course of your day is connected to, and has an impact on, everyone else through the universal web of interconnectivity. The energy and impact of your choices affects the web in ways you cannot begin to fathom. Your energy—even when you think it is inconsequential—is a vital part of the web, and your vibrations affect countless others.

With every day that you live and breathe, your energy affects the whole. For this reason, you must ensure that your personal energy vibrations are of the highest frequency and purest quality by remaining aligned with your inspired soul-view.

This universal web or field of Source energy not only connects everything, but it permeates everything everywhere—all of the unfilled, bare space in the universe—the air between you and this book, for example. You may have previously considered blank space to be nothing, mere empty space. Instead, consider it as an energy substance—a creative energy plane, an intelligent force, a Divine presence, a medium that carries energy and creates. Call it whatever you want, but the energy inherent in this blank space connects your being to everything else, and is all-powerful. Its power is greater than any of the human demands we could ever place upon it. Far more than empty space, it has the ability to respond to your thoughts, emotions, and beliefs as if they were magnetically drawn into this realm.

Your connection to the universe is not an insignificant point. The universal energy plane where our souls originated is the parent, if you will, to all of our souls. It is at this unseen energy level that we're connected to each other. We are intrinsically all part of the same consciousness. As you live with certainty you will develop an ever-increasing sense that every person, animal, and creature on the planet is part of your soul-family, an interconnected aspect of yourself. We all live interconnected within the unseen, just as we are linked in our Earthly proximity.

Part and parcel of this theory of interconnectivity is that every other human is as significant and as powerful to the universe as you. Your soul is connected to the soul of every other being—all of whom have a unique purpose and are equally important. We are all connected by our energy, the very energy that comprises the universe. Our interconnectivity becomes more than just an abstract concept when you consider that the energy of your thoughts, actions, beliefs, intentions, and aspirations travels immediately through the universal web of interconnectivity, and affects how and when the dominoes fall in the lives of countless others.

Oneness

For the purpose of this book, Oneness is a spiritual idiom describing the transcendent unity of every aspect of existence within both the spiritual and Earthly physical realms of the universe. It is the belief that everything is emanated from Source energy, and as such is all divine and equal.

It's easy to understand that you are connected to Source energy, but you also must realize that if you are connected to Source energy, everyone else is, too. You share the same origin and have a direct connection to everyone else—even someone you may perceive as your worst enemy. From this enlightened perspective, your ego is weak and powerless.

In a sense, because our souls share our parents—Source energy—with everyone else in the universe, we are essentially siblings with all other humans. Every single person is a reflection of Source energy, and it is from this perspective that we must respect the souls that inhabit each of us (although we may not be drawn to the ego-personality). In a soul sense, we should not be strangers to one another.

Once you embrace the concept that we are all one, all living relatively the same Earthly experience, you will have made a breakthrough in your quest to live aligned with Source energy. Living your life in Oneness and harmony with every aspect of the universe—our fellow humans, the planet, and every tree, animal, flower, stone, or river—should be one of your highest goals.

Our time in Earthly physicality is intended to be *more* about the collective We and *less* about the individual *I* and *me*. The connection between others and ourselves needs to be something we feel, not just something we attempt to intellectualize. You must know, accept, and feel connected to your own inspired soul-view in a deep and meaningful way in order to feel this greater union.

You've Felt It All Along

Think of your fellow humans around the globe as souls. When you gaze at a sunset or at the moon, consider how many other people are doing the same thing at the same time. You should immediately feel your energy heighten. Now consider this mass of humanity as a single Earthly community connected at the Source. As geographically dispersed and different as your ego may want you to think we all are, you must accept that at the core we are all—each and every one of us—made of the same stuff.

If processing this fact seems difficult, start on a smaller, more intimate scale. Once you're comfortably connected with your inspired soul-view, look at your family members and closest friends through a spiritual lens, and attempt to get a sense of their essence. Think of each of them as a soul. Begin looking at everyone as if they are a part of you, and imagine their essence as being cut from the same cloth as yours. You will naturally find yourself feeling far more tolerance and compassion.

If you still aren't getting it, try this. Recall a time when you have been moved to tears or experienced overwhelming joy as you witnessed someone win an award, scholarship, or sporting event, or accomplished something no one believed possible. That intense emotion that you naturally feel is evidence of your connection to others. Once you have this epiphany, you should naturally have more empathy for others.

To quickly change and soften your perspective on "strangers," begin smiling at everyone you meet. Most everyone will smile back. It breaks open your shell—and theirs—allowing you to feel more vibrant and confident. You begin to feel that you have something important to offer and share. The walls between us begin to fall. Radiating love and kindness, or making someone else feel noticed or acknowledged, is never wrong. Your energy will vibrate higher, and you'll experience more joy. At the same time, I do realize and acknowledge that there are places and cultures around the globe where you may live or travel where offering a smile may not be a safe idea. In these circumstances, it's best to shrink your smile sphere to those whom you know and trust; it will still be a difference maker.

Compassion and Interconnectivity Go Hand in Hand

Truly experiencing interconnectivity comes from having compassion for others. As you progress in your Living with Certainty journey, you'll find that this revelatory approach to life and spirituality makes it far easier to see, feel, and accept that you are interconnected with all of humanity, and to view others with genuine interest and greater depths of love and compassion than you ever thought possible. It's worth repeating that you must be gentle, kind, and compassionate with yourself before you can achieve this with anyone else. As you learn really to love yourself through discovering your purpose and aligning with Source energy, you really learn to love others.

We must approach others and ourselves more compassionately. As you are kind to others, you are kind to yourself—and vice versa. When you truly understand and internalize our interconnectivity, love and compassion will come more naturally and instinctively. When you act with more compassion and fearlessness in your relationships, your energy heightens and you become more of who you are meant to be. By virtue of your strong sense of interconnectivity with all else, you will begin to emanate a love and tranquility that feels good and right. This is the beginning of deep-soul joy.

We cannot experience Oneness when we're harboring feelings of envy, jealousy, or opposition. This is precisely what has led to the proliferation of feelings of isolation and separation. We spend more time trying to show how distinctive and unique we are, rather than attempting to come together through fostering connection and Oneness—yet, conflict and differences tend to dissolve when we embrace our interconnectivity.

Say that you're stuck behind an elderly person in a walker or wheelchair as you are hurriedly trying to walk into a store. Do you feel impatient, or even angry? Take a moment and imagine that this is a beloved family member—would you want someone else to direct negative emotions at them? Of course not. Suddenly, your negative energy begins to dissipate as you feel more compassionate and protective about this stranger and his or her frailties. You may even find yourself rushing to grab the door for this person, when just a moment ago you perceived them as an obstacle or hindrance.

Bias, Fear, and Discrimination

It takes great belief, understanding, empathy, faith, and practice to live with Oneness. To live an unbiased, nonjudgmental life that welcomes diversity you must broaden your perspective to embrace differences

Chapter 8: Universal Interconnectivity

and unique attributes—always remembering that we all emanate from the same Source.

Your perspective is everything. To truly live with certainty, you must treat your fellow humans as the perfect souls they are, and no longer perceive yourself as superior to them. Understand that whether you are the CEO of a multibillion-dollar global corporation, a celebrity, the pastor of your church, or a mom of four children in suburbia, at the soul-level you are no better or no worse than any of your fellow humans.

We are constantly comparing ourselves to others, making judgments that we are somehow better or worse. The simple truth is that we share more things in common than not with our fellow humans. On the surface we look and act differently, but underneath we are fundamentally the same in our Earthly physicality and spiritual interconnectivity.

Accepting the concept of universal interconnectivity into your life is a process of reconditioning yourself until any hint of separateness and superiority disappears. Living with Certainty will allow you to expand your world and begin to experience the global community in a way you never have before. You will come to understand that when you disrespect others, you are disrespecting Source energy. You not only hurt others, but also yourself when you display fear, bias, judgment, or disrespect toward others. Your fears and biases are completely wasted, futile, negative energy.

Understanding and experiencing our interconnectivity has the power to heal wounds. When you embrace your connection and begin to fully appreciate that we are one—one human species fueled by and sharing Source energy—you no longer have adversaries, foes, and opponents. There's no reason for you to feel the need to combat, defeat, or annihilate anyone else. When you lash out at or harm another, you hurt yourself and possibly others through the negative energy and karma you set into motion. Once you understand how you will suffer from hurting another—even if you don't get "caught" in your Earthly life—you should feel compelled to behave differently.

Allow the concept of Karma to serve as your internal filtering system.

It's obvious that humanity on our planet is inherently diverse. But, as you live with certainty, you will find that our similarities are more pronounced than our differences. This isn't to say that you shouldn't be discerning about differences. Each one of us is a unique individual, different from everyone else. While you need not be friends with everyone, it's imperative for the creation of peaceful life on our planet that you begin viewing others from a place of respect, understanding, empathy, and compassion. Let your mind find similarities first, rather than hone in on differences.

Some people tend to fear those who are different than them. They feel far more comfortable with the known than with the unknown. If this describes you and you want to change, you can make the effort to expand your perspective by exploring and embracing other cultures—through food, music, games, dance, language, holidays, entertainment, and art. Read books, surf the Internet, watch travelogues on television. Do whatever you can to begin to open yourself to a broader point of view.

This can be an exciting and rewarding part of your journey. Try frequenting restaurants that serve cuisine from other cultures. Study the history of the food before you go. If you have the resources, travel to new destinations for an authentic taste of local culture and lifestyle. Learn about the destination's history, geography, and government. The gap between people exists only because it has been taught and fostered. It stands to reason, then, that Oneness can also be taught, nurtured, and made real.

Loneliness

So many people, despite being surrounded by family, friends, and coworkers, still experience feelings of loneliness, separation, or a desire to withdraw. It's when people feel disconnected from Source energy that they experience feelings of loneliness and despair. You may feel this way because you're not living with the universal interconnectivity for which your soul is longing.

While there may be times in your life when you feel small and unimportant, you must remind yourself of your significance within the universal web of interconnectivity. There never exists a time when you are insignificant or unimportant. Your life impacts the energetic workings of the entire web at all times. If you were born into this world, you belong. It's that simple. You are only alone when you dismiss the constant accompaniment of Source energy.

Make a Way

Developing our innate sense of interconnectivity with our fellow humans and nature will improve life and the future of our planet. Mere tolerance is not enough—we must celebrate this diverse planet. We must be open-minded, charitable, understanding, and compassionate if we are to live the lives the universe always intended for us to live. There is no more time to waste. Others may not be as blessed as you are—we are all on different journeys—but compassion becomes a natural outgrowth of experiencing universal interconnectivity, along with a desire to serve and give. There is much to be shared with the greater world through your benevolence and deep-soul joy.

Imagine how much better you could feel—and how much better you could make others feel—if you didn't have the sense that you are in this alone, but felt instead that your burden was shared, and you were unconditionally supported and loved. This is the significance of universal interconnectivity. With it, we can transform the world.

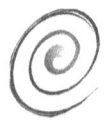

CHAPTER 9

Meditation

*"Meditation helps you to grow your own intuitive faculty.
It becomes very clear what is going to fulfill you,
what is going to help you flower."*
—Osho

IF YOU DO NOTHING ELSE in this book, you should commit to a meditation practice. Meditation is an imperative spiritual practice, powerful and purifying. As you live with certainty you must take the time to self-center—and meditation is your most powerful tool for doing so. It heightens your awareness, penetrates to the tranquility of your inspired soul-view, encourages the experience of universal interconnectivity, and incites the inspiration for aligning with your purposeful authenticity. Meditation facilitates your encounter with higher states of consciousness while enriching your life's journey, and spills into every subsequent moment of your life.

Meditation is a self-directed mental discipline that can help you access a realm far beyond impulsive thinking. The practice of meditation has entered the mainstream, and different types serve different purposes, including relaxing the body and calming the mind, developing awareness, and entering a transcendent state of consciousness. Combined with breathing and mindfulness, meditation is a significant part of the spiritual journey, and plays a key role in moving you more quickly toward the life the universe always intended for you to live.

You may have dismissed meditation as too esoteric, unnecessary, or out there. Meditation is not a religion. There is nothing to fear. Meditation practice can help you build a spiritual foundation—a practical, powerful, and productive goal for anyone who wants to experience more joy, peace, and purpose in life. Meditation is the antidote for the chaotic, desensitized Earthly world we live in, and can serve as your window into another dimension or energy plane. With just 20 minutes a day spent in a pure state of stillness and awareness, you can change your life and come to a deeper understanding of your inspired soul-view. The more you meditate, the more you'll gain a sense of the expanse and mystery of the universe, and the love it has for you.

Meditation and Your Physical Health

Research continues to demonstrate that meditation and other relaxation techniques can have positive effects on our physical health at a deep, cellular level. The range of its positive effects is partially due to increased brain activity in the calmer, left prefrontal cortex, the part of the brain that produces positive feelings and lowers levels of the stress hormone cortisol. This release decreases the negative effects of stress, mild depression, and anxiety, while producing feelings of well-being and tranquility. Meditation also lowers anger levels, and acts as a supplemental treatment for depression, heart disease, and social-anxiety disorders. Activity in the amygdala—where the brain processes fear—is also reduced.[5]

Meditation's numerous physical health benefits include the following: enhanced immune functioning, increased serotonin production, increased exercise tolerance, reduced respiratory rate, strengthening of the heart, improved concentration, deeper levels of physical relaxation, decreased muscle tension, reduced oxygen consumption, lowered blood pressure, better post-operative healing, enhanced blood flow, reduced viral activity, enhanced energy and strength, reduced cholesterol levels, slowing of the aging process, and improved endocrine system function.

Where to Begin?

There are dozens of excellent, detailed books, along with a myriad of instructional DVDs and classes that focus solely on meditation and its history, purpose, and benefits. Rather than focus on detailed technique, this book will provide a brief overview to get you started, while focusing more on the importance and benefits of meditating as you live with certainty. It will be worth your while to acquire a book or DVD on various meditation techniques so that you can choose the one that is right for you. My own starting point was Transcendental Meditation.

Meditation does not require that you become an expert, only that you consistently practice. It is an exceedingly simple journey that must be entered into with an open mind and no expectations. You will reap benefits, even if consciously you don't immediately notice changes. While the results may initially be subtle, they'll be there from the very beginning. Don't put pressure on yourself or try to force anything—just begin with the knowledge that you will experience benefits.

No matter your physical circumstances, career, or relationship status, you are capable of meditating and finding your center, and infusing yourself with the spiritual strength to co-create the life the universe always intended for you to live.

Following are basics for beginning a meditation practice:

- Create an inviting, quiet, peaceful area where you can be alone. It should have good energy for you, and be devoted solely to meditation. Fill it with objects that have meaning for you and make you feel good—flowers, mementos, photographs, candles, small statues, incense, or other objects of personal significance.

- Choose a time to meditate that will work for you daily without the interruptions of phones, emails, television, or kids. Commit to a timeframe and then stick with it. I strongly recommend meditating for at least 20 minutes per day. In the beginning, however, it may help you to set an egg timer for a shorter time. You can gradually increase the duration as you become more comfortable.

- Sit comfortably in an upright position with your back straight. Be still, without fidgeting. Take several deep breaths to begin relaxation. Keeping your focus on breathing deeply is an important aspect of meditation.

- Concentration is required to quiet your mind. Relax. Breathe deeply. Keep your mind open, aware, and in the moment. Don't try to achieve anything. Go easy. Find your stillness and then allow. There is nothing to force, nothing to expect. Trust that the benefits will be there for you, just as they are for everyone.

- It may help to close your eyes and repeat a mantra, a word or phrase that resonates within you. You might try the Sanskrit mantra, *Om Namah Shivaya,* or something more familiar that has personal meaning, such as *I honor the Divinity that resides within me*—or even simpler, *I am love.* Your mantra can be anything that allows you to focus and still your mind.

- Expect your mind to wander. Remain aware so that you can immediately notice these thoughts. Refocus on your breathing and/or your mantra, and quickly bring yourself back to your center. Thoughts will cross your mind just like fluffy clouds passing overhead. You need only to notice and release them. Don't be distracted by your thoughts during meditation. Instead, tell them, *Not now—I'm doing something far more important right now.* When you come out of meditation, maintain that openness in your mind for as long as you can. Try not to allow thoughts to creep back the second that you stand up.

You may be a bit uncomfortable with the unfamiliar silence of meditation, but it is nothing to fear. Silence is essential to the experience, as it creates the open space into which guidance and messages can emerge. You must deliberately surrender on a daily basis to this more gentle state. As your body and mind relax, your spirit will gain the space and silence to surface. In short order, you'll find your time in the meditative state to be addictive, and your body, mind, and spirit will at times yearn for this softer place.

Remember, the time you spend meditating each day will have a positive impact on you, right up until your next session and beyond. Trust that your meditation is changing and helping you, even if the progress and results seem subtle. I can assure you that as soon as you stop, you'll find yourself returning to old patterns and behaviors. At first you may have to be persistent, but over time the practice will become effortless.

Accessing Your Inspired Soul-View Through Meditation

Meditation is a powerful way to care for your spirit because it creates a still, clear, peaceful, empty space in your mind into which the richness of your inspired soul-view and purposeful authenticity can emerge. Your soul lightens and rises as it is freed from the dense noise and static of thoughts, feelings, and activities. You'll quickly realize that the "sense of nothingness" that people use to describe meditation is actually *everythingness*. You align with the egoless spiritual plane that's filled with knowledge of everything, including the insight you need in order to live the life the universe always intended for you to live.

Never lose sight of the fact that the subtle knowledge of spirit can only emanate from the purity of the here and now. This alone should be enough reason for you to still yourself and meditate. For anyone whose thoughts run rampant to the past, future, and everywhere except the here and now, the experience of meditation is truly transformational.

Meditation allows spirit to become your dominant guiding state. This time spent communing with your inspired soul-view is pure renewal. It releases unwanted stimuli, leaving you more relaxed, aware, and clear-minded and with the necessary space for your inspired soul-view to emerge.

Almost immediately you will feel the effects and enjoy the benefits of meditation. This new, calmer state from which you live will become your new baseline. Remember meditation is required not only to achieve, but also to sustain this new state. It costs nothing—and is an essential aspect of discovering your deep-soul joy. Begin today.

CHAPTER 10

Your Purpose and Purposeful Authenticity

*"There are two great days in a person's life—
the day we are born and the day we discover why."*
—William Barclay

CAN YOU TELL ME who you are and why you are here without deferring to labels that have been placed upon you by others? It's easy to answer, "I'm a father" (or student, banker, teacher, Democrat, American, college graduate, and so on), but using labels like these doesn't answer the question of purpose in any profound or meaningful way. It is much harder to answer the question by assuming purpose.

Do you know what you want? Do you really believe you can have what you want? If the answer to either question is no, you have work to do. And, if you answered yes to both of those questions, you should also naturally and quickly be able to answer the following questions: What are your deepest desires? What are your passions? What excites you? What do you most treasure? What are you most grateful for? How do you want to serve? What brings you great joy? What do you want to learn? What are you most proud of? What must you accomplish before you die?

To live a life that is an expression of your purpose, the answers to essential questions like these must come easily to you, and align with one another.

Breakout Understanding

When you embrace your authenticity and discover your essence, you will achieve *breakout understanding,* an epiphany that makes the purpose of your life crystal clear. Breakout understanding inspires and motivates you to do the work and take the action that is required for you to live the life the universe always intended for you to live. From here, there's no turning back.

What Is a Purpose?

We are all born with a specific purpose, the reason for our existence. You too have a specific reason for being that leverages your own specific interests, skills, and abilities. It's important to realize that you may not have just one purpose for which you have entered into Earthly physicality to complete, but rather a series of roles and tasks that will build upon themselves, raising you to the next level of service. Everything that you do, conceive, and accomplish—all of your thoughts, beliefs, and actions—that are in alignment with your inspired soul-view have a snowball effect, and become integrated into the development of who you are now, and who you will become.

Without question, identifying your calling can be difficult. Though we are complex beings with a variety of interests, know this: Where your calling is concerned, there will be no mistaking it. Following a calling causes you to feel a certain joyful purpose that you experience no other way—you feel connected, authentic, vital, energetic, engaged, enthusiastic, and grateful.

Your purpose is not merely your ideal vocation—or desired paycheck. Rather, expressing your purpose is life-encompassing. This includes professional pursuits and vocation; spiritual inspiration and enlightenment; health and wellness; thoughts and beliefs; actions; physical environment; financial circumstances and resources; love; family and relationships; and hobbies and recreation—all of which must be aligned in support of the creation of the life the universe always intended for you to live through the expression of your purposeful authenticity.

Even if you're presently uncertain as to what your purpose is, this knowledge is within you, just waiting to be discovered. This is not an elusive, tricky, or difficult journey—your purpose longs to be encountered and expressed.

Chapter 10: Your Purpose and Purposeful Authenticity

Purpose and Vocation

Your vocation is a primary route to self-actualization. The most joyous people are so intrinsically aligned with their work that they consider it their primary channel for expressing their essence. What better way to share your gifts with the world than through your vocation? When aligned with your purposeful authenticity, your work releases all of the inspiration, creativity, feeling, and energy you need to co-create the life the universe always intended for you to live.

Your soul longs for the opportunity to live its purpose on Earth. When your vocation or daily activities are an expression of your purposeful authenticity, you'll feel compelled to seize and utilize every possible moment to engage in this purposeful activity. Vocation that expresses your purposeful authenticity actually heightens your awareness, bringing you naturally into the here and now. This allows for more inspiration and creativity. When you are fully present and engaged, you're utilizing your highest abilities, rather than wishing you were somewhere else.

This isn't to say that there won't be frustrations—they are an inevitable part of every aspect of life—but despite frustrations, your vocation feels like a "labor of love", an apt phrase used to describe efforts that are fueled by your soul's highest purpose.

Purpose and Ego

Following the path of purpose requires that you relinquish your egotistic self, because your soul's needs for its own development might be diametrically opposed to your ego's desires. Spirituality and egotistic self-indulgence simply do not go together.

It takes time and thought to finally understand that the Earthly fulfillment of your inspired soul-view is a very different life path than merely fulfilling your goals for your bank account. The journey begins the moment that you start being authentic and stop trying to be powerful and influential. You must let go of your ego's mistaken notions of what will make you happy.

Of course, that's easier said than done if you have spent your whole life toiling away so you can buy that mansion on the hill or that red Ferrari. These possessions do not express your purpose. You must learn to distinguish between these incompatible impulses as you maintain your authenticity, balance, and soul-center. Living with certainty will teach you to escape this trap.

Purpose Preventors

Deciphering your purpose on the planet is the real and significant work of your life. This is how humans bring peace, love, and joy into this world. One of the best predictors of happiness is whether a person feels his or her life has purpose. Without it, people tend to feel unsettled and insignificant.

Perhaps you know you're not happy and not living the life of your dreams, but you aren't really sure what you want or where to begin. When you find yourself blocked like this, it's a sure sign that it's time for inner work. Self-exploration is required for you to begin living joyfully and authentically. Your identity—the way you see yourself—is one of the most powerful driving forces of your life. It drives your actions and creates people's perceptions of you.

If you're unhappy, take stock. Who are you and what do you stand for? What have you done—or not done? What are the triggers causing you to feel this way? Do you fear rejection if you reveal your true self to others? Have you edited and stifled yourself to the point that you no longer know where your passions lie? What have you tried to change without success?

It is far more difficult to move through your life pretending that you are someone you are not, than to embrace your authenticity. With authenticity comes peace, but it takes courage and self-confidence. Like so many people, you may have spent a lifetime repressing your passions and gifts in order to fit in, be accepted, measure up, or be conventional. As you were growing up, you may have valued security and love more than a life of authenticity. Now that you have gained some level of maturity, you find that you can't deal with the unrest and anxiety of living out of alignment with your essence.

In trying to evolve singularly in an Earthly state, what have you grown to deny or dislike about yourself? Consider whether you have expressed interests that other people have discouraged you from pursuing. Inhibition and embarrassment have no place in this journey. You cannot censor, edit, or stifle your dreams because of preconceived notions or external pressures.

As you move through life, it is inevitable that other people will try to define and pigeonhole you, particularly if you don't define your own life. You needn't waste time worrying about what others think, or looking outside for consent or approval. No one else knows how you should live your life. Everyone has different dreams, and different definitions of joy and success. What really matters is that you unleash yourself, the very best of yourself. Aligning with your purposeful authenticity doesn't require anyone's approval except your own. It's important to remember, however, that purposeful authenticity is a life of integrity. Alignment with Source energy is a higher, more evolved spiritual state. It's not a license to run wild, or to be a slave to hedonistic pursuits.

The fear of being watched and judged can have an inhibiting effect on you, so stop worrying about what others think. You must learn to disregard the stares, observations, or judgments of others. Even when you are being watched, don't change—remain authentic and unruffled and carry on with your business. Much responsibility is required to be a unique individual.

What Is Purposeful Authenticity?

Purposeful authenticity refers to the Earthly expression of the essential purpose of your inspired soul-view. It is the most profound form of self-actualization. Your purposeful authenticity encompasses your highest endeavors—your intended service to the planet. Never lose sight of the fact that through universal interconnectivity the successful expression of your purpose affects the Whole. By living with purposeful authenticity, you are in alignment with Source energy and constantly receiving divine guidance through signs, signals, symbols, and synchronicities. When the choices you make in every moment vibrate positively with you and cause you to feel good, this is a sign that they are aligned with your soul's purpose. You are taking a purposefully authentic approach to life in which your individual authenticity, dreams, and passions are not only expressed, but are also celebrated and savored.

Accepting the concept of Oneness and universal interconnectivity by no means implies that you should compromise your unique attributes. It does imply, however, that somehow, your purpose is to be of service to others. Your job is consistently to be your most authentic self while recognizing that intrinsic connection to all else.

To pursue your purposeful authenticity, to follow your calling, is a choice. If you ignore the calling, you'll be frustrated and disappointed, always wondering, *What if?* You may even equate your lack of fulfillment or courage with having failed. Interestingly, the urges and signs propelling you toward soul-view–aligned action do not disappear, despite your repeated refusal or denial, until you have acknowledged, comprehended, and processed their message. The universe won't let you off the hook easily; Source energy wants you to make your deepest contribution for yourself and the universe.

Purpose and Success

Success is the attainment of a life that expresses your purposeful authenticity. Deep-soul joy naturally follows. It's that simple. Once you discover your inspired soul-view, you may be surprised to discover how simply you are able to live, all the while experiencing deeper levels of happiness and joy than ever before. Regardless of how you have defined success for yourself up until now, you must understand that you will only enjoy true, lasting success and deep-soul joy when you have the courage to unearth and embrace your purposeful authenticity. As you live your purpose, consciously allow your feelings of success to feed your joy—and allow your joy to feed your efforts toward further purposeful success.

Discovering Your Purposeful Authenticity

You are a one-of-a-kind masterpiece, whether you're currently expressing your inimitable distinctiveness or not. Your journey to purposeful authenticity requires that you confront and accept every aspect of yourself. What about you is unique and different that could be used to offer something to the world that it's never before seen?

As you live with certainty, much will be revealed through guidance from Source energy about your purpose, and the course of action that's required. What does it feel like to receive Source guidance relative to your purpose? As stated before, it can come as hunch, inspiration, instinct, intuition, feeling, emotion, or urge, and appear through signs, signals, symbols, and synchronicities. Noticing it requires vigilant wakefulness.

To discover your purposeful authenticity, you must meditate and pray and regularly find time to be introspective, contemplative, and still. You must also follow your instinct and be extremely sensitive to your flow. When you feel energized, eager, excited, joyous, passionate, and fortunate, follow those feelings. Keep your expectations in check—don't expect that one day the discovery of your purpose will hit you over the head. While that could happen, it's likely to be far subtler, yet still unmistakable. You will feel it with certainty.

Taking Action: Creating a Life that Expresses Your Purposeful Authenticity

The task of finding your passions and calling can seem daunting. Still, you should have nothing but optimism and faith in this journey to discover yourself. While the universe is, and always will be, mysterious, you are not a mystery to the universe. It knows everything there is to know about you. Your soul wants to tell you what you need to know. Relax into the journey. All that's required is your intention to find answers—and your belief that you will be successful.

Since your Earthly life is intended to be a creative, inspirational expression of your purposeful authenticity, you must think about what statement you want to make. Once you do this, your every dream, thought, belief, action, inclination, principle, and ideal must work in alignment with this statement and purpose.

By now, it should be clear to you why awareness is the first Energy Enabler. A life of spiritual enlightenment requires that you open and awaken. You will not discover your purpose through mere thinking or study—you must fully accept that what you are seeking is inside of you at this very moment. You merely have to uncover it—not create it.

While in a state of motionlessness and tranquility, ask what purpose the universe has for you. Meditate on this—it's the most powerful tool you can use to pursue this end. Think, pray, and meditate on the following questions:

- What are your innate preferences and tendencies?
- What were your earliest leanings and loves as a child?
- What urges and hunches have repeated themselves over an extended period of time?

The answer will only come through awareness of what you are sensing and feeling. From this state of motionlessness and tranquility, inspiration is free to unfold with clarity and immediacy. You just have to remain aware of what comes to you via thought, hunch, and feeling—one moment your mind may be still and blank, and the next you may have an urge or a deep feeling of knowing.

During meditation and prayer, ask for guidance and inspiration in discovering your inspired soul-view and purposeful authenticity. Answers may be revealed through intuition, signs, signals, symbols, and synchronicities. Before beginning meditation, ask the question, *How can I center my life on this passion?* Begin prayer by asking Source energy for guidance and help in creating the ideal circumstances to enable you to live your purposeful authenticity. You might ask, *Please help me to bring forth the ideal people and circumstances to do this thing; I know what I want, I now require your help in making this happen.*

Visualize yourself engaging in activities that you really love until you experience positive feelings of joy and fulfillment. Do this several times every day. You need to be able to see clearly these things in your mind's eye. When you know what you want, this will become easy. By spending time thinking more about the things that make you feel good, you begin to bring them into your experience.

Grab a folder, and start filling it with pictures and images torn from magazines and newspapers that make you feel positively stirred inside—happy, curious, and intrigued. These are things that you would like to have as a part of your life. You should be able to place yourself into these images—actually be able to see yourself engaging in these activities.

Once you have a full folder, make a collage of these images on a wall or piece of poster board. Visual cues can help make the images of what you want more vivid and real in your imagination. Make time to sit and contemplate these images frequently. See where your thoughts take you, and how things start to come together.

The amount of work required to redirect your life may be immense. However, when this work is aligned with your purposeful authenticity, it comes naturally. Once you discover what really matters to you, you'll find yourself driven to do it, finding every spare moment to apply yourself. This is when your creative juices flow and great things begin to happen. This is the first step in the success process—to do what you love, to find your rainbow, to be enthusiastic about your life and your work.

Instead of thinking in terms of jobs, take the time to ponder—in a far broader sense—the things you most enjoy doing. Any time you go through a transition, you must allow yourself time to regroup, rejuvenate, and reassess the direction of your life. Accurate self-assessment is crucial to becoming clear about what you want. This includes evaluating your strengths, favorite activities, responsibilities, and passions, as well as the things you avoid, dislike, and dread doing. Once you have established a direction in accordance with your inner voice, it may be helpful to bounce ideas off of your objective inner circle or mentors. These individuals can probably provide valuable information about how you and your strengths are perceived.

You may also find the following very basic tips helpful as you begin your journey to discover your purposeful authenticity:

- Create a "purpose journal" in which you document all that will be required from you as you begin the transition to a life of purposeful authenticity. Include whatever hard and soft skills will be required; what contributions your family members may need to make during the transition; practical day-to-day challenges that you'll likely face, and so on. Write freely and without inhibition about your strengths, special skills, passions, talents, values, and motivations. Write about your answers and reactions to the following subjects: How disciplined are you? What are you really willing to work for? How motivated and ambitious are you? What are your intentions? Are you currently leveraging and utilizing your strengths? How do you feel about your potentiality? What is your purpose? Are you living authentically? If not, what's stopping you?

- Clean house by eliminating those aspects of your life that you have been tolerating, but which add to your anxiety, lack of fulfillment, or stress. If you cannot completely eliminate these things, how can you lessen their impact on your daily life?

- Contemplate comforting thoughts and things that bring you feelings of contentment, fondness, and joy. When you were a child, innocent, naïve, and full of hope, what did you dream you would be like as an adult? Did you dream of the life you are now living? Would you want the person you are now to have been a role model for the child you once were? Locate and listen to your inner child's voice. Keep your child-like goodness, optimism, and wonder alive.

- Seize the moment to pursue anything big or small that carries meaning, or that you have longed to do but have put off because you were too busy. It's by no means a waste of time to dive into any feeling, sensation, thought, activity, or pastime that makes you feel engaged, purposeful, and contented. If you have always wanted to take a course or class to further develop your strengths, natural passions, or hobbies, now is the time.

- Reach out to others. No matter how bad your own situation seems, there are always others who have it worse. Help them. It will make you feel useful and better. Any time you give love, you are awakening your true self.

- Release self-imposed limits that have been dictating what you think is achievable and possible for yourself. Think only about further defining your purpose, without putting a cap or limit on your dreams.

Practical Considerations

Transitioning your life to revolve around your inspired soul-view can be complicated. You may have too many responsibilities at this point in your life to do anything that seems impulsive or uncertain. As you awaken to your purpose, part of you—the logical, cautious you—will want to run. Our essence pushes us to reach higher while our ego-personality metaphorically encourages us to curl up in the safety and security of the familiar. On your journey to purposeful authenticity, things such as commitment, discipline, boldness, courage, patience, faith, and tolerance for chaos and complexity will be required. You will undoubtedly experience challenges that test your conviction and your faith. You may experience doubt as to whether what you are unearthing is the real thing, the calling that's worth enduring risk, chaos, and upheaval. There is no circumventing the fact that discovering your purposeful authenticity—who you are, what you want, and why you are here—takes hard work and courage.

For years, you may have pushed your calling's deepest yearnings to the back of your mind, not wishing to deal with the complication and fear that would ensue if you followed your passions. Unquestionably, some sacrifice for you and your family—possibly including tremendous upheaval—may be required, especially if your current inauthentic life is miles from where you are headed.

While you may be fully aware of your unique gifts and passions, you may not know where to begin when it comes to making a living, or how to share your gifts in service to the greater world. Don't despair. Very few people step seamlessly into their dream without toil and effort. Lighten your load by living with awareness in the here and now, and focusing on what needs to be done today. Don't fret about the future. Irrespective of the hurdles that seem to stand in your way, adopt the perspective that every aspect of this journey is intended to help you learn, develop, and expand your horizons as you co-create the life the universe always intended for you to live.

From a practical perspective, here are some of the challenges you will likely face as you begin to change your life:

- The momentum of your current, non-soul-view–aligned life path, possibly including your steady paycheck, will be slowed or even completely halted. This may require that, for a while at least, you continue working in a job that is not your ideal situation, but nevertheless pays the bills and takes care of your family.

- Similarly, your various involvements and commitments may need to be halted if they do not align with your new path. Extricate yourself from any activities that you have somehow been roped into that don't feel good, right, or purposeful.

- Once you have gotten practical about what changes will be exacted, you have to communicate clearly with everyone who may be impacted. Be prepared to carry an extra load during the transition, knowing that the ensuing lifelong experience of deep-soul joy will be worth it.

- If you don't feel good about something, or if you feel any doubt, stop. Sleep on it and see how you feel in the morning. If you're still not sure, give it one more week (if that's possible or practical) before making any decisions. Whether you wait 24 hours or a week, listen to what your emotions and feelings are telling you. The right decision will feel good, and allow you to feel relaxed and at peace. The wrong decision will cause you to feel tense, and to experience doubt. Begin taking small steps forward by making inspired soul-view–aligned choices at all times.

Identifying Your Passions

In the context of living with certainty, passion is the all-consuming, strongly felt affection, energy, motivation, warmth, emotion, and

Chapter 10: Your Purpose and Purposeful Authenticity

enthusiasm that emanates from your soul about things for which you have tireless concentration and focus. Passion is high-octane soul fuel that inspires commitment and excellence. Your passion centers on the things that:
- You are interested in
- You pay attention to
- You are curious about
- You stay informed about
- You read about
- You participate in
- You love to do and wish you could be paid for

What does passion feel like? Your passions are a result of interests and talents that fill you with positive emotion and joy. As you pause to consider your passions, you may experience a sense of anxiety if nothing immediately comes to mind. This is where awareness is needed. You may need to think of the word passion differently and in more practical terms. Your natural talents, strengths, and passions are revealed to you through your everyday life. Stop expecting a lightning bolt. Start noticing the activities and the interactions that bring you pleasure. What comes easy?

Questions for Contemplation and Discovery

Your purpose and passion represent the creative extension of your soul. Without a doubt, you have the ability to bring your purposeful authenticity into Earthly form. To begin this process, ask yourself essential questions and write your answers in your journal. While your passions may presently seem elusive, relax into the thought that they are inside of you right now. All you have to do is peel back a few more layers. The following questions may help you toward this end:
- What brings you joy, pride, and satisfaction?
- What makes you enthusiastic and excited?
- What engages you to the point that you lose track of time?
- When do you feel at peace?

- What did you love to do as a child?
- What makes you feel talented and confident?
- What activities and thoughts are you engaged in when you experience the strongest connection to others, or a pull to use your gift to be of service to them?
- When do you have the most energy?
- When does inspiration and creativity seem to strike?
- When do you feel that you are making your most significant contribution?

You have to know what you are passionate about and what you want if you're to make deliberate choices that will serve as the building blocks of purposeful authenticity.

Faith and Confidence

Pay attention to your inner voice, intuition, instinct, gut feelings, and emotions. Rarely will they mislead you. There is no need to question whether you can be successful in your soul-view–aligned endeavors. You'll no longer question your commitment or competencies. Rather, you'll feel uniquely qualified and supremely confident. Inspiration and opportunity will emerge. Action aligned with your inspired soul-view is destined to be fruitful and successful.

Deep-soul joy and the creation of the life the universe always intended for you to live will be achieved as you deliberately choose to develop skills, participate in activities, and share your innate gifts with the world through pursuits and endeavors that cause you to feel joyous, passionate, and enthralled. This is how you will achieve your potential and greatness. The activities of your daily life must be a meaningful labor of love if you are to create the life the universe always intended for you to live. Your passion is a guiding light; run toward it.

CHAPTER 11

Your Internal Instruction System

"Your mind knows only some things. Your inner voice, your instinct, knows everything. If you listen to what you know instinctively, it will always lead you down the right path."
—Henry Winkler

SOURCE ENERGY IS THE ALL-KNOWING, omnipotent, creative energy, and intelligence of the universe, perfect in its infinite goodness and power. It graces our lives with its immeasurable wisdom and affirmations. Best-selling spiritual author Gary Zukav describes this guidance as follows: "Our nonphysical assistance comes from ranges of nonphysical Light that are higher in frequency than our own. The intelligences that assist and guide us ... are of a higher rank in creation than we, and therefore, can provide us with a quality of guidance and assistance that we cannot give to each other."[6] This is very true, and it is the precise nature of this higher vibrating energy that makes it incumbent upon us to live with certainty, thereby enabling the heightening and purification of our vibrational frequency so that we can better align with Source energy.

None of this grace means a thing, however, if you don't learn to know yourself. We have firmly established that living an inspired life requires that you become sensitive to energy. Developing sensitivity to your personal energy rhythms and vibrational frequency is essential if you are to utilize the innate, remarkable human attributes intended by Source energy to assist and guide you.

At any time or place, and in a manner that no one can ever take from you, you will be able to look inward, touch your soul, and garner the guidance—the only guidance that exists—directing you toward the life the universe always intended for you to live. This knowing should infuse you with unwavering hope, self-assurance, and self-reliance.

Learning to Discern

Through living with certainty, you learn to strengthen your energetic link to your intuitive abilities. Heightened sensitivity to your energy vibrations will result in enhanced discernment faculties. You will naturally become better at discriminating between what truly matters and what doesn't. This is seeing the world from a far broader perspective. You will be able to discern whether you are vibrating at a high or low frequency level. Recognizing these deviations in your energy will allow you to redirect your choices and how you feel. As you set a new baseline of experience and feeling, variations can be immediately detected and remedied. This will place you squarely into the dynamic flow of life and your spiritual power frequency. As you learn to read energy vibrations about people, places, choices, and circumstances, your overall resonance will become more positive, further aiding the transformation of your life for the better.

Your Physical Center

When doubt or negativity creep into your experience, your chest and solar plexus become heavy and tight. This should immediately sound alarms that you have fallen out of alignment from that which is good, right, authentic, and compassionate. It's important to be aware of vibrational fluctuations, whether small or large, that happen throughout your day, and to manage them so that you may remain in alignment with the flow of your spiritual power frequency. When you feel bad, your chest is tight; when you feel good, it's relaxed and open. The solar plexus, a network of nerves located in the abdomen behind the stomach (also known as the "pit" of the stomach) provides similar guidance. When you move from a circumstance that doesn't feel good into a place of authenticity, compassion, and flow, your chest and solar plexus will loosen and relax in a way that is affirming and reassuring, and any tension will dissipate.

Learning to Listen to You

When you experience a nudge to do something based on how you feel, it is not logic-based; this is a spiritual nudge. It is essential that you learn how to tune in and trust the internal guidance that comes to you through your internal instruction system. This internal knowing moves your soul-based transformation forward, and is what brings significant, enduring change into your life.

Emotions and Energy Rhythms

Your emotions are the part of your Earthly consciousness that reflect your interpretation of events, thoughts, and self-talk. Emotions are forms of energy—some make you feel good, and some make you feel bad. Your emotions are a guidance system that allow you to track the pace and pulse of your thoughts. This very real feedback allows you to redirect your actions so that your personal energy vibrations remain at a pure, high frequency.

Our emotions point us directly to aspects of ourselves, particularly wounds that we need to heal. When this happens, you should acknowledge the pain. Feel it, contemplate it, and then move on. When you're unable to understand where a current emotion is coming from, objectively dial back to a time in the past when an experience caused you to feel similarly. As you process the root causes of your emotions and confront the triggers, you'll need to focus more on alignment with what you have control over, and less on what is attempting to control you. Over time, as you repeatedly feel the pain and thoughtfully contemplate the root cause, emotions begin to lose some of their force. Out of repeated emotional experience, you are permitted to heal.

People often live from states of emotional negativity because they get used to feeling a certain way—even if it's dysfunctional. They run the same negative thought loops over and over in their minds, and carry baggage from old, painful experiences. Sometimes, these negative thoughts of the past grow to epic proportions and become far worse than the original event. Some people even go so far as to manufacture present day drama, because they have conditioned themselves to believe it's normal to feel this way.

Turmoil and pain are relative. If they occur often enough, you can become desensitized, struck numb by repeated physical or emotional pummeling. These experiences condition you to close down physically and mentally, the opposite of what's needed spiritually. Know that you have the power to enable or disable these energies with respect to your spirit. You can begin to heal from within, just as you can heal from without.

Whether the drama and accompanying emotions are real or manufactured, they create dense, low-vibrating, static-filled energy. Not only this, but if you allow yourself to be consumed with thoughts of the past, you sacrifice awareness of the here and now, along with your ability to remain open to guidance and messages from Source energy.

Peaceful, balanced emotions are necessary to prevent static, and permit you to remain in the flow of your spiritual power frequency. You cannot have emotions cluttered with drama and static and still expect to feel good, or to clearly receive Source energy's guidance and messages. It takes a mindful, proactive, disciplined effort to remain centered, balanced, peaceful, and calm as much as possible. Keeping any negative emotions and energies in check will help you to dwell from your soul-center.

Intuition

Intuition is the ability to understand, know, or sense something immediately without conscious reasoning. Through intuition, we receive guidance from a more intelligent, spiritual realm of existence. This is guidance you must follow.

We are all born with intuition, a gift that can assist us in every choice and decision of our lives. Think of it as a sixth sense, as it doesn't require physical senses to be experienced. All too often, however, we move forward based on our conscious mind, not factoring in or honoring the intuitive feelings that can keep us out of harm's way, inspire us, and let us know whether or not we are living in expression of our purposeful authenticity. Without question, acting upon intuition takes faith.

What does intuition feel like? It may be a feeling of attraction or revulsion; hope or fear; confusion or clarity. It could appear as a thought or visual image, a hunch, a dream, a compulsion to do something, or a flash of deep knowing.

Our intuition is one of the most reliable means we have for living in alignment with Source energy and our inspired soul-view. As with most of our spiritual abilities, awareness creates the space from which intuition emerges. Without awareness and openness, you can miss subtle, intuitive messages. When you are aware and open, intuition guides you naturally in accordance with your highest self. You will most strongly experience intuition when you are open, truthful, and adaptable.

Approach the development of your intuition with the intention to develop it. Once you know what it feels like, you'll look for it and be more at ease acting upon it. As you examine the meaning of seemingly random events, you'll begin to hone your intuition. As you become increasingly aware and sensitive, you will realize that you are constantly receiving guidance.

Instinct

Similarly, instinct is the way people or animals naturally react or behave below the conscious level, without having to think or learn about something. It is an undeniable feeling—a gut reaction—that you should allow to direct your choices and decisions to go or not go. Let your instinct be a guiding force. Operating in alignment with it reliably helps you remain clear-headed, courageous, and certain. Instinct helps you get in touch with your gut, and less in touch with your ego's desires.

Internal Instruction System

By now, we've well established that encouragement, support, and guidance from Source energy comes to us through a variety of ways: emotions, intuition, and instinct, as well as through signs, symbols, signals, and synchronicities. This is your internal instruction system at work. Your internal instruction system exists within you, allowing you to receive universal guidance intended to help you express your purposeful authenticity. These feelings represent the voice of the real You—the compassionate, loving, enlightened, and infinitely wise *soul-You*. Your feelings, particularly intuition, are the key driver of your internal instruction system because they are the most reliable means of sensing whether you are on the right track. The beauty of your internal instruction system is that it allows you to feel inspiration, guidance, and messages long before your thought process ever kicks in—providing that you remain open and aware.

As you contemplate the various aspects of your life—mind, body, spirit, purpose, vocation, relationships, pleasures—take note of how you feel inside. Do you feel light and joyous, or dense and anxiety-laden? Are you happy and calm, or are you nervous, tense, and uneasy? This exercise can help you to develop awareness of how your energy changes as you think about different things. It will also help you to identify the areas of your life that are in need of work. The goal should be to feel peaceful, joyous, and enthused about each area of your life.

When you feel open, enthusiastic, and compelled to move in a certain direction, move that way. Conversely, when you feel shut down, anxious, and unsafe about moving forward, don't move. You should make decisions based on the choice or option that keeps you feeling aligned with your inspired soul-view, spiritual power frequency, and deep-soul joy. These choices may not be the easy choices, but emotionally and energetically they will feel good and right.

Listening to your internal instruction system is a lifelong commitment and a choice you make every day. This guidance comes to you with certainty—it feels wise, sure, and peaceful. Once you develop a strong connection, surrendering in full faith and trust to this source of guidance will naturally banish all muddle, turmoil, anxiety, and trepidation—along with the need to allow your ego to dominate. But it also requires that you develop awareness and perceptual "muscle power." Some messages and guidance may push you clearly in a certain direction, though doubt may cause you to pause, not knowing what your next move should be. All you need to understand is that the right decisions, choices, and actions feel right and "fit" where you are in your life. Even if the work required, or the perceived obstacles to a certain course of action seem overwhelming, don't get caught up in worrying about the *how* of the future. Instead, stay attuned to your vibrational level and go with your gut.

You should understand that you won't at once receive all the answers and guidance that you'll need for the rest of your life. It doesn't work that way. Messages are often subtle. Try to remain vigilant in listening for them at all times. You may suddenly feel mildly stirred or unsettled. While divine guidance often appears in the form of an urge or compulsion to do something, it is often with an intensity that can seem quite mundane and ordinary.

Occasionally, these spontaneous urges may guide you to do something that you normally would not do, or may even perceive as risky. Again, if it feels purely right with no conflicting feelings or energy, follow the urge. You may later realize that doing that one thing made all the difference in your path. This may be something as simple as making a call, sending an email, driving a different route, watching a specific television show, or not attending an event. It could be anything that you say, do, or think. The key is to follow your gut, and take the inspired soul-view–aligned action that feels good and right. Always listen to your gut feeling, even when there is no rational reason to do so.

As you become more confident in your intuitive abilities, some of your anxiety about life—such as what's next, or whether you will make the right choices—begins to dissipate. While listening to this voice will never steer you wrong, ignoring it can lead to pain. You must never disregard the feelings that are intended to guide you toward your purposeful authenticity and inspired soul-view–aligned action. Hearing and acting upon these feelings and inner voices allows you to move forward with full faith, confidence, and certainty, knowing beyond any shadow of doubt that you are co-creating the life the universe always intended for you to live.

And remember—always take time to express gratitude to the universe when you receive important guidance and information.

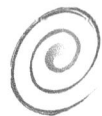

CHAPTER 12

Inspiration and Creativity

*"In my dream the angel shrugged and said,
'If we fail this time, it will be a failure of our imagination.'
And then she placed the world gently in the palm of my hand."*
—Brian Andreas

CREATIVITY IS NOT just for children, artists, or advertising executives. It's for everyone who wants to live an inspired life of purposeful authenticity. Creativity, inspiration, and enthusiasm are divine gifts that we are intended to use to manage, focus, guide, and instruct our own energy and efforts. Our creative abilities allow us to act on our inspiration as we create both intentionally (consciously) and unintentionally (subconsciously). Because you have a soul, you've been hardwired to have all of the creativity you'll ever need to co-create the life the universe always intended for you to live. This creativity and inventiveness is held within your inspired soul-view, and is intended to be applied to and made manifest in your Earthly life.

So many people have said at one time or another, *There's not a creative bone in my body.* Relax, because this isn't true. While some people may have more developed artistic abilities than others, particularly as it relates to business or professional creative applications, we're all connected to and graced by the inspiration of Source energy. And we all have the ability to express our purposeful authenticity. This is only a matter of following our emotions, inspiration, instincts, and intuition.

Living with Certainty and Creativity

Your creative internal voice is your inspired soul-view speaking to you.

As you live with certainty, you will experience inspiration in a way you have never before known. You will become infused with passion and optimism. You will develop a more inquisitive and questioning nature.

The key to manifesting the life the universe always intended for you to live is to remain open to whatever creative expression is revealed to you through your inspired soul-view. Then take action according to the inspiration, imagination, and creativity that flows. There is no ceiling for a soul. There are no grades given for expressing your soul-view. Through the inspiration of your soul-view, you will naturally gain the self-assurance, passion, and motivation required to forge ahead.

Engage Your Imagination

Through your imagination, your inspired soul-view connects with you. If you are not achieving what you want, consider that it may be due to a failure of your imagination. Creativity can rescue you. The ability to use your imagination, to think and see beyond the obvious and predictable, and to envision connections that others may not see—this is creativity. To be truly creative, you have to be open and receptive to your intuition, instinct, emotions, hunches, and randomly appearing events.

We are all capable of using our imaginations; we use them each time we need to initiate action or solve a problem. However, relatively few of us consistently and fully engage our imaginations in the co-creation of our lives. The happiest and most successful people consistently utilize and leverage their creative abilities to realize what they want. Remember, the great discoveries we admire, and the accomplishments of others we stand in awe of, started with a kernel of an idea or a spark of imagination. Thinking big—without boundaries and limits—is the key to developing your creativity.

Give yourself a chance to use your imagination in order to figure out your vision. Follow your internal instruction system regarding which of these ideas holds the greatest potential and most opportunity, and then map your plan. This is the beginning of the process of making things happen.

Ask "Why Not" Rather than "Why?"

Want to be stagnant? Stuck in the mud? Consider it done if you are someone who closes your mind to new ideas. Rather than live a life of limitation, try new things—dream and strive. Greatness comes from not allowing society to inhibit your creativity and authenticity, quell your uniqueness, or dictate constraints. If you think that you're just an average person, or that there's nothing special about you, then you don't know yourself and your gifts well enough. You have not yet discovered your inspired soul-view.

When you're sleeping, do you dream? Well-adjusted, well-rested individuals have dreams that stick with them, inspire them to action, and can forever change them during their waking hours. Dreams provide great impetus for creativity. Ideas can develop from seeds planted in dreams—things that you may never have considered while awake. Never disregard your dreams as meaningless dribble. When you awaken and recollect a particularly interesting or creative dream, write down the particulars and mull them over.

Create and Invent Out of Nothing

The creative thinking process enables us to conceive new goals, new behaviors, and new action plans. And it is this very creation, toil, labor, and inspiration that lead to the expression of your purposeful authenticity and the experience of deep-soul joy. Your creative expression represents your uniqueness and your personal attitude. When you are inspired, you feel dynamic and self-assured. Inspired people aren't afraid to experiment and test their ideas or inspiration. If one thing doesn't work, there are always more approaches or ideas to try.

Creative Blocks

The time to summon your creativity is when you are naturally experiencing joy and enthusiasm. This is when focus, intensity, and genius show up. If you have a nimble nature when it comes to thought and subsequent action, you can change course quickly when inspiration strikes, or when intuition redirects you. You may not have wings, but you can fly in your mind. Give yourself permission and believe in your innate ability to do this. Let your imagination carry you as far as you can possibly dream.

Set aside time specifically for creative thinking and dreaming. Just taking a few minutes a day may be all you need to jump-start creative habits. If you find this difficult, step outside of yourself by imagining how others see you. What could you do that might surprise them? Continually asking questions like this can provide the spark you need.

If you find yourself creatively blocked, you may need to change your environment. Are you surrounded by clutter, noise, or other distractions that may be blocking your energy and creating static? You may benefit from a clean, simple, quiet environment that helps to get your spiritual creative juices flowing. Note, however, that you will fall out of alignment with Source energy and the flow of your spiritual power frequency if you darken your energy and pollute your body through substance abuse in order to summon the courage to achieve new dreams or smother old, broken ones.

Awareness and Creativity

It's easier to think deeply and tap into your creative abilities when you are calm, peaceful, and happy. It's essential to give your mind periods of stillness through meditation, or other pursuits that bring you to a state of motionlessness and tranquility. Intentional, soul-view-aligned creation thrives on keenly focused awareness. Hear what others are saying. Take in your environment. Soak up warm, loving interactions with others.

Meditation may inspire your most significant inspiration. As you clear space for your soul's inspiration to emerge, your intention is understood by Source energy. Your heightened awareness is primed to receive messages of inspiration and insight. When inspiration strikes after meditation, hear it, trust it, and act upon it.

Creativity, Youth, and Humor

Think back to your childhood. You could amuse yourself for hours pretending, playing make believe, and daydreaming. It felt good. As you got older and consequently took on more responsibility, you may have become overly disciplined and serious. However, you needn't lose those beautiful, creative traits of your youth. By rekindling the child within you, you breathe life into your creative side. Children see and experience the world with such wonder. Can you even recall when you last felt this way? Try to take yourself back to that place. Where did that ability go to slow down and really take things in?

Joy and humor are interconnected. Don't lose your lighter side. Humor should always be a part of our lives, not just our childhood. Life allows for an abundance and profusion of joy. The more able you are to stay connected to your lighter side, the easier it will be to maintain, develop, or redevelop your creative abilities. Lighten up, have fun, live!

PART III

The Living with Certainty Lifestyle: The Energy Enablers

*"The religion of the future will be a cosmic religion.
It should transcend a personal God and avoid dogma and theology ... .
It should be based on a religious sense arising from the experience
of all things natural and spiritual as a meaningful unity."*
—Albert Einstein

The core aspects of your daily life, including your spirituality, thoughts, emotions, actions, and beliefs, all emit energy. When high-vibrating and pure, this energy enables you to align with the flow of your spiritual power frequency. To some extent, your energetic vibrational level and present life circumstances are the result of deliberate choices you have made. Every choice, intention, and action either heightens or lowers your vibrational frequency. It either brings you closer, or takes you farther away from your inspired soul-view; and either puts you in, or takes you out of the flow of your spiritual power frequency. The quality of the energy you expend is the reality of the experience you receive in return.

Many people compartmentalize or draw lines between the different aspects of their lives—there's the Monday through Friday life of career, school, family commitments, and running a household; Saturday is for entertainment and recreational pursuits; and Sunday, a day of worship and introspection. This is the wrong approach to Earthly physicality, since every aspect of your life and energy overlaps and is interconnected. Where you go, your soul goes. When you live a compartmentalized existence, you shortchange your potential, waste precious time, and live outside of the ways of the universe. The Living with Certainty approach closes the gap between your spirituality and daily life by enabling you to more authentically and purposefully navigate through life's inevitable challenges by engaging in behaviors and activities that are supremely gentle, aligned, compassionate, loving, and altruistic.

Your soul has one clear dilemma where your Earthly physicality is concerned—your ego-personality's attempts to dominate your soul's voice. To resist this opposition, the Living with Certainty lifestyle consists of seven mind-body-spirit categories that provide direction for moving through life while keeping your energy vibrations at a high frequency level. If we all lived with certainty, we could immeasurably elevate the collective energetic vibrational level of our planet, resulting in waves of joy.

This book's 65 Energy Enablers provide an adaptable and practical approach to spirituality, emphasizing that there is no separation between spirituality and Earthly life. Each essential principle for living in accordance with Source energy stands on its own as an honorable approach to life—but taken together, they comprise a powerful, practical philosophy for elevating your spiritual energy.

Each of the 65 tenets requires considerable effort, if not mastery. You may find the integration of these practices into your life to be seamless and easy, or they may require a vast change in thought, beliefs, and lifestyle. Daily practices or reactions that used to require little thought or effort might now take more time, awareness, patience, and effort—and, it's precisely this discomfort that benchmarks your transformation.

How you incorporate the Energy Enablers into your life is ultimately your choice, but I suggest that you initially focus on the areas that feel comfortable to you. Don't overwhelm or frustrate yourself. Take baby steps in the beginning. You may find it practical to begin with the "spiritual energy" enablers and, once mastered, move consecutively though the remaining sections. I recommend that you first read through the entire book, and then begin the program as a whole. The companion *Living with Certainty Discovery Guide* will help to fuel your efforts, whichever method you choose.

It's important that you read and contemplate these topics. Expect to feel uncomfortable at first, but know that this feeling is only temporary while you assimilate this new approach to life.

If you feel yourself becoming overwhelmed, simply slow down and focus your time on developing your awareness through stillness and meditation. As you regain your center, you can once again focus on the Energy Enablers. As your energy consistently aligns with a higher-vibrational frequency, you'll experience authentic empowerment to transform your life in a way that feels at once natural, inspired, passionate, purposeful, peaceful, and joyous.

What works for me will work for you. The Energy Enablers will make it possible for you to establish and integrate spiritual and energetic force and momentum into every aspect of your life.

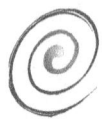

CHAPTER 13

Spiritual Energy

"Spiritual energy flows in and produces effects in the phenomenal world."
—William James

ENERGY IS AN ESSENTIAL ASPECT of your spiritual journey. Though it is largely imperceptible to us, physics teaches that every aspect of our universe is comprised of energy. We are surrounded by energetic transmissions, and while we cannot see the vibrations, we can feel them.

Our spirituality encompasses the level to which we have welcomed Source energy into our lives and created a life that is the fullest possible Earthly expression of our inspired soul-view and purposeful authenticity. When we live a spiritual life, we are immersed in loving, compassionate, purposeful energetic transmissions.

The energy of the Earthly and spiritual dimensions vibrates at different rates or frequencies. In his best-selling book, *One Last Time*, psychic medium John Edward has the following to say about energetic vibrational levels: "All of us—we in physical bodies and those in the spirit world—are made up of energy expressed as atoms and molecules spinning and vibrating at certain speeds. The energy of spirits vibrates at a very high rate, while ours goes much slower because we are in physical bodies. How we bridge the gap dictates how well communications traverse these two dimensions ... . For spirits to come through, they must slow their vibrational rate of energy ... I speed mine up. Communication is what happens in that space in between."[7] He goes on to say that he raises his own vibrations through meditation and praying the rosary.

Think of the universe as a web of interrelated strands of energy that emanates to and from everyone and everything. The individual, invisible strands of this energetic web of life constantly vibrate, and extend to each of us. At this very moment, energy is flowing from you and to you through these invisible, yet powerful, strands of energy.

As you vibrate energy to and through this web, you are co-creating your life. Everything exists first in this unseen realm before it's made manifest in Earthly physicality. Think of this intricate energetic web as the incubator or blueprint for every aspect of human life. Your energy affects everything else and you, in turn, are affected by the energy of everything else. Your dreams, desires, thoughts, feelings, beliefs, and emotions are all measurable energies—they emit vibrations that affect the vast, universal web of energy. Your physical world is a partial reflection of your metaphysical world. Energy changes as your thoughts and beliefs influence it.

When your energy vibrates at a high frequency, you feel good, expansive, vast, bright, optimistic, and light, with a strong sense that you're in the flow of your spiritual power frequency. You are more inclined to see the best in everyone and everything. You look at life through a lens of connectivity and love.

The Spiritual Energy Enablers of Love, Self-Awareness and Self-Love, Compassion, Service, Allowance and Surrender, Revelation and Enlightenment, Acceptance, Prayer, Peace, Silence and Solitude, and Communing with Nature are essential building blocks for enhancing your spiritual life and transforming your spiritual energy to the highest vibrational frequency.

1. Love

*"There is more hunger for love and appreciation
in this world than for bread."*
—Mother Theresa

Love is an unselfish, warm, tender feeling of affection and attachment. Love is high-vibrating energy, feeling, and force, and is the most significant element in our Earthly lives. It is the "master" frequency—

the optimal energy vibration we should strive for at all times. Love's pure intentions create the highest frequency energy vibrations. It is a transformational energy in every respect.

When you give love, you project the highest frequency energy out into the universe. It works every time. This pure energy does not involve material things such as wedding dresses and diamond rings—rather, it involves complete connection, compassion, service, and acceptance. Love connects us. As you live with deep-soul joy, you live your life in and from a state of love. And when you approach every aspect of your life with this high frequency, loving approach, you elevate the energy of everything you do, allowing it to be felt by everyone with whom you interact.

Love allows us to learn about ourselves in profound ways; it also teaches us much about other people. But it requires effort. Our ego-personalities create problems for us in the realm of love by adding static to, and lowering the frequency of, this otherwise pure energy. We set limits around our ability to love, when there should be none.

More love in the world could positively change every aspect of human existence and experience. Love will be the basis of your spiritual quest—love for yourself, others, Source energy, nature, and our planet. Love, along with compassion, forgiveness, Oneness, gratitude, and altruism is the highest spiritually energetic level to which you can aspire. As you live with certainty, you will begin to transition to a far more loving and compassionate foundation for relating to the world and everything in it. A surefire shortcut to enjoying the bounty of living with certainty is to allow yourself to feel love in everything you do. Through love your sense of universal interconnectivity and compassion are exponentially increased.

2. Self-Awareness and Self-Love

"What is necessary to change a person is to change his awareness of himself."
—Abraham Maslow

A beautiful life includes having a healthy respect for your self. With healthy self-esteem, you can withstand setbacks and defeats, accepting them as isolated incidents or transactions that are part and parcel of dealing with daily life. They don't shake you to your core, or let you waste time dwelling in the negative. Source energy knows who you are, where you are, and what you need. Your job is to remain in alignment with this highest and purest of energy. A healthy self-esteem can help you do this, and as you express your purposeful authenticity, your self-esteem will rise.

Sadly, too many people suffer from feelings of personal inferiority. They place excessive focus on defeat, as if it represents who they are or their future potential. Low self-esteem is the root of much negativity and skewed thinking in the world, and it can be difficult to overcome.

If you have battled with feelings of self-loathing, worthlessness, guilt, and shame, now is the time to make peace with yourself. You'll never move forward until you do. It is essential to the Living with Certainty process that you confront your true nature. Be grateful and accepting of the authentic you. This is an essential step in your spiritual journey. Again, I remind you that if you were born, you belong. The world awaits your unique contribution as you become unbound.

Perfection really isn't a human quality, and none of us will ever achieve it. We can only do the best we can at any given moment. Maya Angelou once said, "You did what you knew how to do and when you knew better, you did better."[8]

Don't know where to begin? If you lack feelings of self-worth, you have to change your thinking. This takes internal fortitude, belief, and discipline. You must awaken the courage to face and relate to your deepest fears and anxieties. Everyone has unique virtues, as well as unique vices—you must accept both, and embrace who you are. Only you (perhaps with the aid of a therapist) are capable of doing the inner work that will foster healthy self-esteem. In the words of Ralph Waldo Emerson, "Nothing can bring you peace but yourself."

Begin at the soul-level by noticing and honoring your emotions and feelings, demonstrating respect for your higher self. Stay true to the task of discovering your inspired soul-view and purposeful authenticity. A good starting point is to reach out to others. By helping others, you will always make yourself feel better, useful, and of service. Any time you give love, you awaken your true self.

Self Talk

Self-talk is the running commentary in your head, and can include observations, judgments, problems, anxieties, and worries. You must monitor this self-talk in order to recognize when you are being negative or pessimistic with yourself. Any time you find that your self-talk has turned negative, let the thought go, open your heart, and remember that your job is to build a bridge of love to yourself. You can't achieve this by continuously knocking down the foundation.

Be gentle with yourself as you begin this process, which may include changing a lifetime of negative thoughts. It takes awareness to monitor what you are telling yourself on a minute-to-minute basis. If this proves difficult, try changing your tune. Tell yourself that transitioning and uplifting your thoughts is easy, and that you are successfully doing so. Your positive self-talk should outweigh your negative self-talk by a ratio of 10:1.

Self-Assessment and Self-Awareness

Meditation is great for raising your awareness, but you must also take time outside of meditation for serious introspection and self-assessment. Be kind to yourself as you begin this process. Take an inventory of your strengths and soft spots, which reflect who you really are, what you really love and value, what you really require developmentally, and where you really excel. Your strengths are those attributes that you have relied upon to help you move through life. Use them, work with them, and make the most of them.

You cannot live with certainty while operating under false illusions. Accurate self-assessment requires you to be completely honest with yourself without allowing your ego-personality to protect you from your Truth. Through this process of examination and introspection, you will experience great freedom.

While you should feel good about the effort you have put into achieving your goals so far, it may be time to change course if you are not where you want to be. Owning up to what's working in your life and what's not requires going deep, and becoming clear about who you are, what you stand for, and what you want. You must conduct a thorough, honest, and realistic assessment of your strengths, weaknesses, limitations, beliefs, activities, responsibilities, passions, and dislikes. If you are truly to accept yourself, try to view yourself and your life with perspective and objectivity, as though you are a spectator. And remember—it helps immensely to be able to laugh at yourself and your mistakes, and to forgive yourself as you do so.

We all have soft spots. When faced with stress, pressure, or difficulties, we can become different people, barely recognizable to ourselves or to others. Be ready to identify—without judgment—your crazy behavior as crazy, your destructive behavior as destructive, your ill intentions as ill, your mean behavior as mean, and your jealous feelings as jealous. The good news is that once identified, you have the ability to let go of the unproductive thoughts and behaviors that may be holding you back. But first, you must stop ignoring, resisting, repressing, and denying them. This is how you begin to resolve your issues, and release the negative feelings they engender.

Once you become aware of, and familiar with, how your negative actions and behaviors make you feel, the intensity of experiencing them begins to diminish. As you begin to accept these aspects of yourself as part and parcel of who you are, you'll be able to face them while remaining at peace with yourself. These aspects are a part of you that you are here to understand and heal. Stop hiding from yourself; there is nothing to fear. All of this is part of discovering and embracing the soul-You.

Self-Acceptance, Self-Respect, and Self-Love

Doc Childre, HeartMath founder and global authority on optimizing human performance and personal effectiveness, stated, "Ultimately when we learn to truly love and accept ourselves, we'll be able to live well and to love each other and everything we encounter."⁹ Before you can truly experience deep-soul joy, you must first experience self-love and self-respect. They will form the foundation from which you interact with the world.

Welcome the notion that the real you is not your ego-personality, but rather your inspired soul-view. See yourself first as spirit. Your sense of self should be aligned with your inspired soul-view, purposeful authenticity, and potential, as well as with your obligation to spread love and compassion

You have a responsibility to love yourself and embrace your worthiness. You must become your own best friend and biggest fan. You will do this by accepting that at your essence, you are inherently miraculous and perfect Source energy, living in an Earthly body. As you discover your inspired soul-view, loving and respecting who you are and why you're here becomes easier and less complicated. To experience deep-soul joy, to eliminate static and align with the flow of your spiritual power frequency, to generate energy at the purest, highest vibrational frequencies possible, to live the life the universe always intended for you to live, you must love yourself unconditionally.

3. Compassion

"Compassion is the relative spirit of enlightenment; it is reaching out in love to all beings who have yet to realize that they are unborn."
—Drom

Compassion is having deep awareness and concern for the distress of others coupled with a deep desire to relieve it. The pure energy of love flows within you as you observe an aspect of life, a person, or circumstance. Rather than judging or turning your back, compassion causes you to want to relieve others of their suffering. Compassion is the greatest and most powerful bond between you and your fellow humans.

Developing compassion does not require lessons or affiliation with a specific religion; it only requires that you embrace the frail qualities of humanness that we all share. Once you make the decision to live with compassion, it supremely influences how you view the world.

As you incorporate increasing kindness, service, and compassion into your relationships, you will awaken more.

Seize any opportunity to practice tolerance and patience. Your goal must be to live without bias, judgment, or discrimination toward anyone or anything, anywhere at anytime. Compassion should be the most basic of your values.

We're all capable of compassion, yet there doesn't seem to be enough of it in the world. As you live with certainty and weaken your ego's stranglehold, it will become a more natural response. It's not a difficult process to develop compassion, and you will become more compassionate as you embrace the concept of universal interconnectivity. Think of it as taking empathy to a new level. Project with your heart what it feels like to stand in someone else's shoes, and you'll experience an overwhelming desire to help.

The totality of the Living with Certainty approach will assist you in understanding that there is no place for judgment, blame, lack of forgiveness, harm, or hate in your spiritual journey. With compassion, your desire to help and heal grows more powerful than anything—and it becomes a relief for you to allow your judgments, opinions, and negative energy to dissolve in favor of kindness and feeling good.

Compassion should not just be limited to your inner circle or family. It must become your humanitarian approach to every aspect of the world. "Do unto others as you would have them do unto you"—this is the ethic of reciprocity, also known as the Golden Rule. Take this to heart. Compassion requires that you treat everyone, not just those of whom you approve, with consideration. Open yourself and reach out. Compassion begins one person, one interaction at a time.

4. Service

"Strange as it may seem, life becomes serene and enjoyable precisely when selfish pleasure and personal success are no longer the guiding goals."
—Mihaly Csikszentmihalyi

Innate to embracing your purposeful authenticity is the motivation to help and serve others. You finally know who you are, and are assured by Source energy that you have more than enough to share. Your newfound sense of personal fulfillment naturally fuels your desire to extend yourself. Any time you give love, you are awakening your soul. Service enriches and deepens you as it changes your perspective about your relationship with the Earth and your fellow humans. When you shift your focus to include others, and seek to improve their lives, your own growth and enlightenment ultimately benefit.

Begin simply by reaching out to others. Each day, big and small occasions arise that afford you the opportunity to help and serve others. No matter how bad your own situation may seem, there are always others who have it worse. By helping them, you are helping your own alignment. One person's service has the potential to set off a chain reaction that helps many people—also known as the concept of "paying it forward."

Service signals alignment with Source energy and elevates you to the purest, finest realm of energy the universe knows. Once you live with awareness and connectivity, enhanced selflessness comes naturally and the compulsion to share, serve, support, assist, and teach is natural and powerful. You can be an agent of light in this universe—a symbol of love, compassion, and kindheartedness—each and every time you reach out to help. As you do so, you set in motion currents of unconditional love that vibrate throughout the universe.

The notion of service shouldn't be about taking credit or receiving kudos. If you want to test drive how it feels to give without expectation of gratitude and acknowledgment, give to someone anonymously. It feels great. When you truly release the need for acknowledgment, you get more out of it. Consider that the people who aren't grateful or who don't give thanks are often those who need the most love shown to them.

In this lifetime, you are intended to commit to significant service to a purpose larger than your own individual motives. When you show compassion, caring, and love toward people in need, you touch them just through making them feel worthy. Be the light that provides attention and validation to others, and be the one who hears those in need and gives them a voice. An act of kindness or service on your part can change someone's life.

5. Allowance and Surrender

"The tragedy of life and of the world is not that men do not know God; the tragedy is that, knowing him, they still insist on going their own way."
—William Barclay

As you live with certainty, you will sense those times when you cannot control or change your external situation. How novel an approach would it be for you to stop resisting and to surrender instead?

While the mere mention of giving up "perceived" control in order to surrender to a higher power may cause your hair to stand on end, know this: Surrender is an essential aspect of deep-soul joy and purposeful authenticity. Ironically, it is ultimately when we surrender that we experience a greater sense of contentment and freedom. Part of going with the flow is accepting that the joys and travails of your life are intended for your development; they are part and parcel of the life the universe always intended for you to live.

Let's be clear, however, about what surrender is, and what it's not. It doesn't mean that you no longer have to take action. When you surrender as you live with certainty, you make the choice to live from a place of pure faith that the universe is working on your behalf. You submit to Source energy's infinite wisdom, and make the choice to have patience and to go with the flow—accepting and allowing that events and circumstances are transpiring exactly as they should. As you surrender and open yourself to the grace of Source energy, you will receive.

Surrendering frees you from the shackles of your ego. Your well-being and highest good comes when your ego's death grip deactivates through surrender, and you make the choice to renounce the fleeting and temporary aspects of life in favor of that which feels spiritually good and right. You do this because you trust that this is the path that will further your own enlightenment and transcendence.

Up until now you may have felt that you were struggling to swim against the current, rather than with the flow of your life. If you find you have developed a hard edge or brusque exterior, it may be because there is a well of pain you are covering or denying. If you have been resisting dealing with your issues and soft spots, a healthy step forward is to let go of the struggle, and to relax and surrender.

Ironically, you may have felt that not dealing with your pain was the easiest way to move forward, but resistance fights flow and doesn't allow you to deal with situations in a healthy manner, or move beyond them. It is only by surrendering to pain and allowing yourself to experience it that you can diminish it. In this way, you create an openness—a space—to let go. Step by step, you'll reveal your strength of spirit and allow it to become your primary source of energy and direction. You alone determine the amount of static that is allowed to affect your power frequency.

Surrender is essential. It allows you to let go of anxiety, worry, and the need to control. When you are attached to a specific outcome—particularly one that's not in alignment with your inspired soul-view—you are adding static to your frequency. Once you let go of your attachment to outcomes, however, your energy heightens—enabling an easiness that allows you to tap into the flow of your spiritual power frequency. Resistance restricts your ability to align with your flow and to manifest your soul-view–aligned desires.

Your intention to surrender is crucial, because Source energy responds to intention. Once the intention and requisite efforts are firmly in place, you can mentally and spiritually relax and live a life that expresses your purposeful authenticity. Things that you want come about when your mindset is trusting and open, and ready to receive the soul-view–aligned gifts you desire. Once you surrender, your life will be easier. Things will fall into place. This isn't something you can force, but rather something you allow. As you trust and relax, you will reengage with the flow that was disrupted through your attempts to force and control outcomes. Let it go, let it be, and if it is intended for you, you will co-create it.

6. Revelation and Enlightenment

*"Cease trying to work everything out with your minds.
It will get you nowhere. Live by intuition and inspiration
and let your whole life be Revelation."*
—Eileen Caddy

Revelation is the connection to your innermost self that profoundly impacts and naturally inspires you to live a purpose-driven, principled, and honorable life. As you undertake this spiritual journey, you will open yourself to the possibility of experiencing revelation, which will truly alter your life and spiritual state. Revelation is profound. It goes hand in hand with your transformation as you discover that you are so much more—and connected to so much more—than you previously perceived. When you experience a revelation, you will unexpectedly and abruptly know beyond doubt that the disclosure is emanating from an otherworldly source. It is an intense and moving experience.

Enlightenment is an ongoing journey, and takes place naturally as you live with Oneness and in alignment with your inspired soul-view and purposeful authenticity. There is no one right path to enlightenment, and it is never fully attained. There is always another level, and new heights of fulfillment and joy to be achieved. Until our last breath, our lives are intended to be lived in pursuit of fulfillment and enlightenment, which are closely linked. As you become enlightened, you experience the higher, loving, compassionate state of your being. You live with peace, faith, and wisdom, in alignment and love with Source energy. Earthly physicality and ego's grip are loosened. Love and compassion come easily, and what once were perceived as problems become personal growth opportunities.

Gratitude is an essential aspect of enlightenment. As we pursue a life of ongoing development, we must always remember to be grateful for all that we have in the here and now, without being focused on transcending to the next level. I once heard it said that it is better to be a live goat than a dead king because if you are alive, you still have a chance to recover, rebuild, or remake. When we feel and express gratitude, our anxiety and fear weaken, and we are reminded of our universal interconnectivity.

You can only achieve true change in your life when you are growing and evolving, and to do this you have to be present at every moment. And yes, that means feeling and experiencing the highs and the lows, the euphoria and the suffering. You can only grow and enlighten as you become able to discern the consequences of your actions. Those who are truly enlightened experience everything in their lives, while at the same time thinking deeply about how they feel, what they feel, and why they feel that way.

7. Acceptance

"For the most part we humans live with the false impression of security and a feeling of being at home in a seemingly trustworthy physical and human environment. But when the expected course of everyday life is interrupted, we are like shipwrecked people on a miserable plank in the open sea ... . But once we fully accept this, life becomes easier and there is no longer any disappointment."
—Albert Einstein

Acceptance is an important aspect of living with certainty in several respects. First of all, we must accept that we are not in complete control of our lives. There will be bumps in the road. Secondly, we must accept the lives and paths chosen by others if we expect to receive acceptance in return.

The reality of our lives is that we cannot control everything and, therefore, must peacefully accept the fact that ambiguity, anguish, and the unexpected are part and parcel of the Earthly experience. People with whom we interact will not always be consistent, reliable, or truthful. They will contradict themselves to suit their own circumstances, often leaving us to pick up the pieces. Our job is to deal with these things without allowing them to throw us off balance. We do this by living with certainty, despite all that we cannot control.

To co-create the life the universe always intended for you to live, you must be comfortable and steadfast living in an inherently undefined and imprecise world. While living with certainty teaches you how to be certain about your feelings and what you are attempting to co-create, you can count on the strange and unexpected cropping up in your path.

Life is what it is. But remember, every situation, experience, and person we encounter is coming to us as part of the universe's greater plan for our learning and development. Once you accept that you are intended to have these experiences for your soul's growth and development, you can begin to find peace in whatever happens.

As you live with certainty and begin to love and accept yourself more, the obvious next step is to love and accept others more. Just as you crave acceptance, so do others. People are starved for approval and love. They desperately fear being left out, isolated, and embarrassed.

You cannot live from a place of Oneness and universal interconnectivity if you cannot accept your fellow humans. When you are negative about yourself or others, it's contagious. Many of the people around you will catch the negativity bug, so be positive. Time spent critically thinking about others and second-guessing their choices and decisions only creates static for you. Others make choices for themselves that should not be viewed as threatening to you, or as interfering with your own choices. Great freedom comes with accepting this.

When you think of someone and negative feelings immediately arise—perhaps even accompanied by a change in how you physically feel—stop and try something new. Sit for a moment and think without judgment about this person's life. What did you love about this person at one time? What are his or her best traits? What are this person's perceptions of the world that may be causing him or her to act and behave this way? What personal obstacles has this person endured, such as abuse, addiction, or poverty?

As you ask yourself these questions, you will find that contemplating the different paths other people have taken makes it easier to accept who they have become. But remember that acceptance is accompanied by choice—it may well be that if a person generates more static than you can handle, you may have to remove yourself from his or her company.

8. Prayer

"Pray as though everything depended on God.
Work as though everything depended on you."
—Saint Augustine

Prayer is an essential aspect of every religious or spiritual practice, and is considered a direct means of communing with Source energy. A prayer is an act of humble and sincere communion in word or thought addressed to Source energy. It is expressed as an earnest request, or as devotion, confession, praise, or gratitude. The basis of prayer is generally the same as that of visualization, imagination, wishing, and even dreaming—all of which serve to create energy vibrations that are perceptible to Source energy.

The beauty of prayer is that you can do it anywhere, anytime—even multiple times throughout the day. People all around the world pray. You can determine what works best for you, as there are no rules or a single way to pray properly. Your prayer practice does need to be continual—a daily commitment you make as you live with certainty. As it turns out, this is one of the easier commitments you will make along your spiritual journey, since the practice calms and relieves you, while it brings comfort, hope, inspiration, and support.

Prayer has been shown to have positive effects on your fulfillment, health, and joy. There are two types of prayer—directed (praying for a specific outcome or result) and non-directed (requesting no specific goal or outcome). Research has shown that generally prayers are answered more frequently when you don't make specific demands or requests, but rather pray for the best possible outcome—that the ideal circumstances, people, and timing will come together to resolve a particular dilemma. This kind of non-directed prayer can be more successful than directed prayer, although both have clearly been shown to work.[10] This approach takes into consideration the idea that we are co-creators, not singular creators, of our lives.

When should you pray? When times are good or difficult; when you want to express thanks for all that you are and all that you have; when you require guidance, inspiration, transformation, or awareness;

and when you need help discovering your purposeful authenticity or opportunities to serve. You can pray for yourself or for others; for more love, tolerance, or understanding; for help or resolution; or for clarity or guidance to move you toward a course of action. You can pray that people come into your life that can help you move forward in your quest to live the life the universe always intended for you to live. You can offer a simple prayer, inviting Source energy into your life and asking for resolution in line with its infinite wisdom, rather than your own limited wisdom.

You may just pray for relief from pressures and problems until an answer or resolution is brought forth. Regardless of what you pray for, remain aware afterward for flashes of intuition, inspiration, hunches, or signs that are intended to provide answers and guidance. Have faith and remain awake to the answers and direction that will be brought forth.

9. Peace

"Peace: It does not mean to be in a place where there is no noise, trouble or hard work. It means to be in the midst of those things and still be calm in your heart."
—Unknown

To experience peace in your life means that you are free from static and oppressive emotions, thoughts, disturbances, quarrels, anxiety, and stress. This is not to say that difficulties will not present themselves in your life. Rest assured, the universe will intentionally challenge and test your commitment to live with peace in order to boost your own learning and development. As you commit to a peaceful existence, you begin to live from a foundation of tranquility, inner contentment, and serenity. Peace is an attitude, an energy-approach to life. It is the perspective and outlook that allow you to be in the midst of noise or hard work and still be calm in your heart.

For peace to become a way of life, you must first give up judgment, negativity, abuse, and impunity. Finding and maintaining peace in your life is an ongoing challenge. It's easy to remain peaceful when everything is going your way. But how do you remain peaceful when you are faced with turmoil or negativity? This is one of the greatest challenges and tests of our lives.

Any time you begin to feel defensive, angry, or frustrated, retreat to silence and allow yourself the space to choose another response. Try replacing your negative thoughts with a loving thought about the individual with whom you are interacting. Attempt to send the person thoughts of peace and love. This approach will remove your edge and soften your response. You will physically experience your energy heighten as the dynamic of the entire situation elevates and improves.

Do not allow yourself to be adversely influenced by external circumstances; to stand firm and leverage your own power to be an instrument of peace is true enlightenment. When negative energy enters a room, you can make the choice to rebuke it, to say, *Not here, not now, not me.* Too many people have been conditioned to think that negativity is a natural part of our Earthly experience. As you begin to live with deeper understanding and compassion for the human experience, you make the choice to be a channel for peace, stronger and more powerful than the negativity around you. You choose to be the dominant force in your environment, exuding serenity and love. As you consistently maintain an internal state of peace, joy, and love, you will positively change the external energy that surrounds you.

10. Silence and Solitude

"You are never more essentially, more deeply, yourself than when you are still."
—Eckhart Tolle

Living with certainty requires that you make time every day to sit in silence. The advantages of this practice are many. It sorts through the commotion of the day, bringing you calm and clarity. Physically and mentally you allow yourself to relax and unwind as the pressures and stressors of the day begin to dissipate. This is also a very useful practice for externally teaching yourself how your new internal, peaceful baseline should feel. Silence and solitude also help to create that clear space of awareness through which your inspired soul-view can emerge. Stillness allows you to further discover the authentic you—to feel and hear your inner voice, and to experience your own energy, emotions, and intuition.

Stillness should be separate from your meditation practice. Although you can take time for stillness just before or after you meditate, each is a distinct and necessary activity. Stillness allows you to contemplate and pray, while meditation provides an entry point to your soul, or to a separate level of consciousness. Silence and solitude are fertile ground for the emergence of inspiration and intuition. Some messages may be received as a trace indication—perhaps as a bodily sensation, random thought, or feelings.

Our souls are perfect in their peaceful tranquility; however, our ego-personalities pull us out of that place, agitating and interrupting our awareness. All this is part of your ego's misguided effort to feel powerful, and only serves to create dense, low-vibrating energy. Silence and solitude are essential for slicing through this deep fog. It is from a state of motionlessness and tranquility that your world will change.

As you commune with your inspired soul-view, you will gain clarity regarding what really matters and what you really need. From the still state of solitude, you will begin to sense that your beliefs, purpose, and passions are being reorganized or are transforming to something completely different. Irrespective of the depth of the transformation, silence and solitude are tools that prevent you from spinning your wheels and chasing things that are not in alignment with your inspired soul-view and can never bring you true fulfillment and deep-soul joy.

So how do you achieve inner silence and solitude in a jam-packed, chaotic world? Very simply, you sit completely alone without distraction, reading materials, noise, conversation, phones, television, computer, or music. You do absolutely nothing but still yourself in silence. This time alone with Source energy renews and invigorates you. It can help you to locate tolerance and fortitude when you most need it. Physiologically, this place of stillness and serenity is so powerful that it feels immediately healing. You will grow to crave this time as you begin to feel the opening through which all of your other Living with Certainty efforts can emerge and flourish.

The practice of silence and solitude goes hand in hand with learning to live with more awareness. Silence allows you to reconnect with your essence, despite any madness going on around you. It can help you to break destructive behavioral patterns, disengage from damaging emotions, and return to the place of patience, compassion, and forgiveness at your soul-center. When you find yourself becoming angry, excuse yourself and retreat to your silent comfort cocoon. This self-imposed time-out can help to weaken your anger and regain your objectivity so that you can stop being merely reactive. You may be amazed at how quickly anger dissipates once you allow your inner energy to channel your flow away from static.

11. Communing with Nature

*"Earth and sky, woods and fields, lakes and rivers,
the mountain and the sea, are excellent schoolmasters,
and teach some of us more than we can ever learn from books."*
—John Lubbock

Our connection to nature is a significant aspect of our connection to everything else. Nature has a clearing and cleansing effect on our souls. It immediately opens our perspective to our place in the larger universe, and reminds us of the beauty and complexity of which we are a part. The moments when we stand in awe of nature are different from all others. We are moved off the island of ego, bias, and negativity; we are small and humble at the feet of the universe.

In modern day society, we have drifted away from what should be our natural, ever-lasting relationship with nature and the Earth. We have instead turned increasingly toward man-made advances, such as laptops, video games, the Internet, and cell phones. Technological advances improve and enhance our daily lives in many ways. However, when we turn our backs—and our energy—on our innate connection to the Earth and toward a computer screen, for example, it changes the tenor of our relationships with everyone and everything. Clearly, technology has enabled connections between us on a global scale that are staggering, and we are the better for it. But our connection as humans with nature was in no way intended to be only temporary. We need to reestablish a connection to nature to fully appreciate and feel our connection with the universe.

As a species, humans are inherently a part of nature and, as such, need to honor and practice that connection. The fact remains that all sorts of societal pressures have altered our relationship with Mother Nature, along with our connection to each other. Why does this matter? Because when you connect with nature—whether that's sitting under a tree, watching the flow of a mountain stream, or taking in a breathtaking sunset—you vibrate a positive energy into the web of universal interconnectivity. In that moment, you experience true vitality and broadened perspective.

My father referred to being deep in the woods on a camping trip as a *soul bath*. A soul bath happens as you experience natural wonder, beauty, and joy in ways that cause you to feel vital and rejuvenated. You are reminded that there is so much more to the universe than your job and daily commute. You begin to feel ever so slightly different—and better—because your relationship to nature has been reestablished. This may seem like a small change, but it is a crucial one.

If you really want to experience that intrinsic connection with everyone and everything, and to experience the wonder that comes from being in nature, you have to make it a point to be witness to nature's awe-inspiring beauty. Communing with nature through a walk or frolicking in the snow is a natural, simple, and powerful way to find an essential spiritual connection. Strive for quiet, still moments in nature, allowing yourself to stop and take notice of its majesty. If you're city-bound, you can visit parks and zoos, or the Internet can take you deep into a rainforest. A book can whisk you away on an Arctic trek, or a trip to an aquarium or museum can transport you to new environments. Where there's a will, there's a way. No matter where you are, always demonstrate reverence and respect for nature by relating to it with only the highest integrity and intentions.

> **Kristi's Power Enabler**
> *Our spirit doesn't just awaken with our physical birth, nor does it expire with our death. Once you embrace that the single most important aspect of your being is your soul and that this spiritual dimension is always with you ensuring that you are never separated or isolated from Source energy, your life will naturally expand for you in the best ways possible. One of the most loving and comforting aspects of how our universe works is that you have already been provided internally with everything you need to live the life the universe always meant for you to live.*

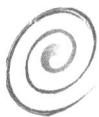

CHAPTER 14

Mind and Thoughts

*"We are what we think: All that we are arises with our thoughts.
With our thoughts we make the world."*
—Buddha

IT IS USEFUL TO DRAW a distinction between your mind and your thoughts. They are not one and the same. Your mind is the thinking and perceiving part of your consciousness that originates in the brain and is manifested in thought, perception, emotion, reason, will, memory, and imagination.

Your life is the sum total of your thoughts. Your thoughts are the lens you use to find the words and mantras you tell yourself every day, and through these words you create your emotions—your optimism, joy, and dreams; or, conversely, your negativity, pain, and fear. Your thoughts carry energy and power. Your current thoughts and beliefs are creating your future, shaping your world, and determining your actions and experiences. You can only change your life by changing your thoughts. Everything in your life—every experience, relationship, and perception—is a mirror of the mental patterns in your head. The inner You creates the outer You.

You co-create your life every day through your thoughts in tandem with Source energy. As a thought originates in your mind and its energy vibrates out to the creative plane of existence, you are entering into the co-creation process. The good news is that it doesn't matter what you've been thinking up until now; the opportunity exists for every one of us to change our thoughts today, and to begin to change our lives for the better.

It's important to remember, however, that you are not your thoughts—you are the essence behind your thoughts. Today, your thoughts may still be closely aligned with your ego-personality. As you begin to live with certainty, however, your thoughts will increasingly become aligned to support the action and expression of your inspired soul-view and purposeful authenticity.

One of the biggest challenges for you as you begin to live with certainty may be changing and controlling your thoughts—how you think, what you think, what you obsess and worry over, and how you allow negative thoughts to create negative emotions. When you are aligned with your inspired soul-view and the flow of your spiritual power frequency, your head is no longer filled with self-defeating thoughts. In general, you will have far fewer thoughts that are negative, toxic, or unproductive. Living with Certainty requires that you become more aware of negative, static-inducing thoughts so that you may transition to positive ones that are in alignment with your inspired soul-view.

Thought Awareness

As you become more aware of how you feel, particularly when you're in a zone of pure, high-vibrating energy and aligned with the flow of your spiritual power frequency, you'll become very sensitive to negativity and its accompanying low-frequency energy vibrations. By carefully monitoring your thoughts, you have better control over your feelings and emotions. When you are truly tuned into your thoughts and the feelings they produce, you'll immediately recognize when you aren't feeling good, and can make the decision to shift your thoughts before they create negative energy. When you get swept up in a torrent of emotional thoughts, take note as soon as possible. Repeat to yourself these words: I'm aware. As you become practiced at repeating this phrase whenever you find yourself lost in low-energy thoughts, you'll begin to build a space between you—the real soul-you—and the opaque, misleading thoughts that serve to lower your vibrational frequency.

Thoughts Create Emotions

Emotion ignites thoughts into strong energy vibrations that have an effect on the powerful unseen. Without emotion, these thoughts are impotent and exist in your mind as mere words. Positive emotions carry vibrations that move you closer to what you want; negative emotions carry vibrations that move you farther away. For this reason, you have to be clear about what you want. Use your thoughts to focus your emotions so that you feel good—and the goal, of course, is to feel good most of the time.

Any thoughts that create intense emotion need to be life-affirming, positive thoughts that create positive feelings. When you have a thought that feels bad, this is your internal instruction system letting you know that a course correction is needed. Very simply, your thoughts are reflected back to you through your feelings—and non-soul-view–aligned thoughts don't feel good.

Your thoughts have a physical impact on your body, as they induce a physiological response. What you do and think creates your moods and even affects your health. Unhappy people spend time dwelling on unpleasant events or interactions, while happy people tend to focus more on positive thoughts. As you live with certainty, you'll become familiar with where your baseline of feeling good should be, and your life will forever change.

Thought Focus

Living with Certainty is your greatest weapon against darkness and negativity. What matters is that you develop the awareness to process and acknowledge where your attention is going, detect any negative thoughts that might arise, and quickly shift to something more positive and productive. Over time and with practice, this will become your habitual, dominant pattern for dealing with negativity. You'll find that you no longer allow your thoughts to become as negative, and that your thoughts will lose some of their capacity to upset you. You have the power to shut them off.

Thought-focus is deliberate, powerful attention on a subject that demands that you remain present in soul-view–aligned thoughts, and ensures that the vibrations you emit to the creative energy plane are consistently positive and in alignment with your inspired soul-view. The Buddhist term "monkey mind" refers to an impulsive, unsettled, erratic, unpredictable, uncontrollable mind that is the polar opposite of deliberate thought-focus.

We all possess the ability to control our thought-focus. Living with certainty is about developing thought-focus that affirms your self, your purpose, and what you want. Co-creating a life that is a pure expression of your purposeful authenticity requires time and awareness. Dwell in abundance, optimism, and possibility; think and believe the best. Once you successfully move the compass of your thought-focus to what feels good and positive, you'll more effectively co-create and attract that which you deeply desire. This requires that you have the clarity of focus to know what you want to the point that you can clearly visualize your desires.

Very positive and very negative emotions carry powerful vibrations. Your life will remain stuck in maintenance mode if your predominate thoughts are negative and lacking in belief. If you spend just 10 to 20 minutes a day, or even every other day, maintaining a thought-focus on what you really want at the soul-level, envisioning things or events as if they have already been manifested, your life will profoundly change. Time spent focused on your inspired soul-view and purposeful authenticity makes you feel good, and powerfully drives your soul-view–aligned action forward.

Creative Thought

You may have told yourself that you don't have a creative bone in your body. The only limit to your potential, however, exists within your mind. By limiting your thinking, you will most certainly limit your reality and, in the process, your entire life. In order to bring your dreams to life, you have to be able to lift the ceiling on any perceived limits, and let the bean stalk grow to heights that you may once have viewed as impossible. Let yourself loose and go crazy with your thoughts—

no boundaries, no limits. Think abundant, feel-good thoughts. Relive positive, joyous times and memories. Consider your thoughts to be the ignition switch that lights your creative fire, allowing you to explore, ask questions, and weigh options. Thoughts allow you to try an idea on for size.

Leveraging Your Mind in Your Spiritual Journey

Your mind and thoughts are intertwined with every aspect of your life and your being, including your spiritual journey. Every day your thoughts impact your Earthly experience. Leverage this power for the good, and focus on utilizing the power of your mind to co-create the life the universe always intended for you to live. Maintain a state of high vibration by focusing on:

- morality, integrity, and principles
- living with honesty and truth
- acting with good intentions
- remaining open
- developing clarity
- making good choices
- displaying courage and confidence
- repeating positive affirmations
- treating yourself and others with good will, kindness, and tolerance
- practicing optimism
- remembering karma
- practicing the Golden Rule

12. Morality

"Let no pleasure tempt thee, no profit allure thee, no persuasion move thee, to do anything which thou knowest to be evil; so shalt thou always live jollily; for a good conscious is a continual Christmas."
—Benjamin Franklin

We can only vibrate energy at an optimal, pure, high frequency when we live an ethical, principled life of honesty, integrity, and morality.

In the long run, you will not get ahead in life when you operate from a place of dishonesty, ill intent, hypocrisy, hate, or disdain. When you act dishonestly, compromise your self-respect, break promises, or hurt others, you create static and lose alignment with your spiritual power frequency, and your energy becomes dense and heavy.

Of course, there are a lot of dishonest people in the world who have profited in the short-run, despite their lack of integrity. However, these are not enlightened individuals who are following a spiritual path. While they may enjoy financial success, their hearts and souls are soiled, and karma will eventually win out. As Tom Peters said, "There is no such thing as a minor lapse of integrity."

Integrity

Integrity is the quality of sincerely and steadfastly being honest, ethical, morally principled, and upright. Living with certainty requires living with integrity—there is no alternative. Your commitment to living with a high level of integrity is part and parcel of living a life that is a pure expression of your purposeful authenticity. It truly affects every aspect of your life, even your health. Everything you do every day, regardless of how large or small, must be done with integrity and pure intention. Many static-inducing behaviors that lower your vibrational frequency lack integrity, such as lying, cheating, stealing, causing harm, and littering. Keep in mind that each time you engage in any of these activities, you immediately reduce your possibilities of co-creating the life the universe always intended for you to live. Integrity doesn't come and go like the tide. It must be a steadfast, essential component of your character. You simply can't operate with a lack of integrity and then expect to align with the supreme goodness of the universe.

As others come to recognize your integrity, you'll attract more like-minded individuals into your life, and will experience far more authentic, trusting relationships and interactions. American Evangelist D. L. Moody once said, "If I take care of my character, my reputation will take care of itself."

High Moral Character and Values

Character refers to your moral constitution, and you must operate from a foundation of knowing what is morally right and what is not. This includes your ethical strength, which is your personal system or code of beliefs, standards of conduct, moral principles, and rules that govern your behavior. To live with certainty is to consistently demonstrate moral excellence and firmness.

Strive to live at all times with moral excellence—behavior that feels good because it's based on right action and thinking. Living with certainty requires moral obligation, and will naturally guide you toward creating a system of values and principles that feel good, right, and are aligned with your purposeful authenticity. Aristotle wisely noted that to enjoy the things we ought, and to hate the things we ought, has the greatest bearing on excellence of character. Living a moral life with a strong sense of right and wrong will serve you well in every aspect of your life's journey.

Consider your values your personal compass for determining right, desirable personal conduct. They are your very own collection of guiding principles that, based on your beliefs of right and wrong, define your actions and control your behavior. Soul-view–aligned action is ethically good; non-soul-view–aligned action can be regarded as ethically bad. When you feel doubtful or unsettled about what you are doing or have involved yourself in, very often it is because there is an inherent misalignment between your values and your actions. What you believe must align with your actions.

Humility

Humility is a human tool for acknowledging that you are a student, always open to learning and development. You can live with purposeful authenticity and feel very good about yourself—experiencing deep-soul joy—and still remain modest in behavior, attitude, and spirit. Pride, arrogance, boasting, and showing off may momentarily feel good to some ego-personality–controlled people, but these are dense, low-vibrating behaviors.

With humility, however, your ego takes a backseat and allows the real You—the soul-You—to receive what you need at every given moment. With humility, you listen, learn, and remain open to moving forward. You can take input and feedback and learn from them. Ego and arrogance do not prevail when you sincerely live from a place of humility, which enables an even stronger sense of universal interconnectivity. You come to realize that admitting when you are wrong, or taking feedback from others, is not a weakness, but is a sign of great strength. Live with humility and in alignment with your own values and let the chips fall where they may.

13. Honesty, Truth, and Facts

*"Each time you are honest and conduct yourself with honesty,
a success force will drive you toward greater success.
Each time you lie, even with a little white lie,
there are strong forces pushing you toward failure."*
—Joseph Sugarman

The truth is steadfast and unfailing. It brings focus and clarity, and eradicates anxiety and confusion. Your truth is empowering. It serves as the foundation for your internal instruction system. You cannot rely on your feelings, instincts, and urges if you haven't been telling yourself the truth, nor can you begin to define what you believe in.

Knowing your truth requires spending time in deep self-reflection. Living with certainty requires that you face the truth about who you are, where you want to go, and where you sit today—and then live in alignment with that truth. Honesty in your Living with Certainty journey is a commitment to truth. As you honor truth, you honor the universe. Living with honesty removes many complications from your life. Just think—no more keeping track of your white lies, or contemplating how to cover your tracks.

Every time you stretch the truth to get your way at work, at school, or in relationships, you lower your vibrational frequency and you destroy your own credibility. Lying is a slippery slope. Once you start lying, embellishing, and stretching—and get away with it—you will be inclined to indulge yourself this way again and again. Even if you don't get caught immediately, the karma you have set into motion will eventually catch up with you. Except for the extremely gullible, everyone around you knows when you are stretching the truth or telling lies, even though they may not say anything. Ralph Waldo Emerson wisely provided a good rule of thumb, "If you would not be known to do anything, never do it."

It is, of course, bad to lie to others—but often, the worst lies are the ones you tell yourself. Your ego would rather lie to you than be forced to acknowledge and face your shortcomings. Yes, it may change the nature of your current circumstances to drop the artificial façade of your life, but so what? The truth is liberating. By being truthful, you encourage others to be open and truthful in return.

Love and truth carry similar, high-frequency vibrations that emanate from a place of good intention and loving kindness. You must take care to never use blunt truths with an intention to hurt someone. Anytime you blurt something out that hurts another, whether it's true or not, you never feel good about it afterwards. You lower your personal vibrational frequency level. Do nothing that harms yourself or others. Remember your karma.

14. Intention
"It's in your moments of decision that your destiny is shaped."
—Anthony Robbins

Your intention is your determination, after careful thought and consideration, to act in a deliberate way. Everything you say or do begins with an intention. Your intentions are at once known to Source energy and are part of the energy equation that co-creates your world. Rest assured—you will be held accountable, so begin with the end in mind. What is the result you are seeking? Let this optimal end result guide you. Your behaviors, actions, and intentions must be in alignment, and should carry a positive intention within a context of value, purpose, and compassion.

As you live with certainty, your intentions become reality as results begin to manifest. Intentions have both direct and remote effects. Strong intention, combined with persistence, is a powerful formula. You alone can change your life—and even the world—by exercising the correct, soul-view–aligned intention. In any given situation, decelerate and ask yourself, *What are my intentions here?* You must answer this question with an authentic resolution that fills you with energy and optimism. Today, make it your intention to live with certainty, to experience deep-soul joy, to express your purposeful authenticity, and to align with your spiritual power frequency.

15. Openness

"It's amazing what ordinary people can do if they set out without preconceived notions."
—Charles F. Kettering

Openness is a place of faith, and with it comes feelings of freedom, peace, security, and joy that result from knowing you have placed yourself in the flow of Source energy. Everything you need—people, resources, circumstances—will enter into your experience at just the right time.

It takes courage and commitment to stay open to whatever comes your way. Openness helps to eliminate static-inducing doubt, fear, anxiety, and uncertainty from your energy, and clears the way for signs, signals, symbols, and synchronicities to appear with more frequency and regularity.

Release yourself from the pressure of feeling that you must provide all the answers, and instead become the one who asks questions. Stay interested in learning more, and seek to understand rather than jump to conclusions and judgments. Be curious, interested, aware, open, and hopeful.

A spiritual journey requires an open, adaptable, and curious approach to life. Be willing to modify your approach to make it suitable for a specific situation or changed circumstance. Interpreting the significance of events, and the various forms of universal guidance and their implications, requires the ability to recognize and make sense of nuance.

Go with the flow with full faith in your intuition—rigidity will not work. As you live with heightened awareness about your environment and how you are feeling, you see and observe more. At times, you may make what seems to others like obscure connections between specific events. So be it. A true spiritual journey is at times emotional, expressive, and inspired. With a flexible and flowing mind, you will see things that a spiritually unaware, logical mind might miss or dismiss. You must tread outside of the confines of logic and reason, and instead be open to the vastness and mystery of the universe and your inspired soul-view.

Your goal must be for your outer shell to be translucent, and in no way blocking your spirit. Openness must become your approach to life, and the faith and trust that emanates naturally from living with certainty will enable you to remain open to what may come. It's easy to settle into a daily routine of just going through the motions, completely unaware of the guidance surrounding you. However, living with openness requires releasing conditioned or programmed responses to events and encourages you to expect the unexpected. With openness, nothing is off the table as a possibility.

Challenges and painful times tend to foster openness. As our senses are heightened, we become more open to lifting our periscope from examining the minutiae of our daily lives to considering essential questions. We gain perspective and realize that there are more important things to worry about than the trivial things that normally consume us and fill our days. During these times, synchronous events serve to provide reassurance, and bolster our faith that we are on track and doing the right things.

Miracles can unfold where there is openness. We become aware of, and begin to contemplate the power of signs, signals, symbols, and synchronicities. We experience our universal interconnectivity and realize that our existence is affecting every other aspect of the universe. We discover and experience our inspired soul-view. Openness is where our possibilities exist.

16. Clarity

"Clarity of mind means clarity of passion, too; this is why a great and clear mind loves ardently and sees distinctly what he loves."
—Blaise Pascal

It should be obvious to you by now that living with certainty requires clarity; you have to be very clear about what you want. As you live from your inspired soul-view, clarity intensifies and strengthens your efforts to maintain a high vibrational frequency level. With clarity, you have no doubt about your life's purpose and potentiality. You live with assurance that every aspect of your life—mind, body, and spirit—is aligned with your purposeful authenticity and Source energy.

Clarity is a life free of clutter and distraction. You're aware of how your energy feels and, therefore, what is right for you. It becomes less of a struggle to co-create your life because you know exactly what you are trying to achieve and are working in alignment with Source energy. How much easier would your life be if you were consistently clear about what you wanted before you took action? Clarity of thought, feeling, and belief should precede action.

To have clarity you must slow down and contemplate the various aspects of your life from the perspective of your inspired soul-view. This helps you to maintain an open space into which inspiration and truth can enter. As you live with certainty, you live with faith that you will receive just the lesson you need, exactly when you need it.

17. Choice

"Whenever I make a choice, I will ask myself two questions: What are the consequences of this choice that I'm making? And will this choice bring fulfillment and happiness to me and also to those who are affected by this choice?"
—Deepak Chopra

Many aspects of your present life circumstances and corresponding energetic vibrational frequency are the result of your personal choices. The decisions you have made have co-created your life. It may seem that there are aspects of your life that you have not consciously chosen to experience. However, your every decision has, in fact, co-created your present circumstances. An essential aspect of Living with Certainty is accepting that you are accountable and responsible for your every choice, action, thought, feeling, and belief—all of which can and do co-create your life.

How do you develop the ability to keep the big picture in perspective while making choices and decisions that very often are based upon limited information? You gather and study all the facts and information possible, and then engage your internal instruction system. Stillness and meditation are helpful, because they create the space for clarity and inspiration to emerge.

Trust your senses by always choosing in the direction of your instinct and feelings. The right choices feel good and align with your direction. They open your solar plexus, relax your chest, calm your mind, and make you feel open, peaceful, and expanded. This feeling of openness and expansion aligns you with the flow of your spiritual power frequency. Uncertainty and doubt are signs that something is wrong, or isn't right for you. When you feel bad, choose again. Wrong choices usually result from using only your intellectual faculties, without engaging your emotions and soul. Wrong choices and ill intentions cause you to shut down, close up, and contract.

Each decision you make helps to create your life. Choices and decisions made in the midst of a busy day may seem insignificant or innocuous, but they can have considerable impact on how your life unfolds. Every choice you make redirects the energy of your life.

You can't control every aspect of your life, but you can choose your thoughts and attitudes. You can choose to view unfortunate circumstances as learning opportunities. While negative events and circumstances befall you from time to time, you have the power to choose how you react, to elevate your circumstances, and to manifest your dreams. Armed with the power of your internal instruction system, you are never stuck and never have to settle.

18. Fear, Courage, and Confidence

"You gain strength, courage and confidence by every experience in which you really stop to look fear in the face. You are able to say to yourself, 'I lived through this horror. I can take the next thing that comes along.' You must do the thing you think you cannot do."
—Eleanor Roosevelt

Living with certainty is impossible when you are frozen with fear. If you are afraid to be yourself, you are fearful of living authentically and will find yourself just trying to fit in or appease others' perspectives and opinions, with no regard for your own purposeful authenticity.

Embrace the fact that life is a journey full of transactions—some easy, some more challenging. We have to muster courage and fortitude to conquer the bumps in the road. How you react to these bumps is what matters—this is where the healing, growth, and learning take place. Living with certainty requires you to look fear in the face without allowing it to derail you. Instead, you must acknowledge and feel the fear or self-doubt, and then move through them. This is where the growth happens; this is where confidence originates. When you know you have to move through an event that has aroused your fear and anxiety, it's immensely comforting to know that in doing so, you remain aligned with your purposeful authenticity and spiritual power frequency. Confidence comes from knowing that you cannot lose because you are living your purpose, and Source energy is directing your course.

Fear

What exactly is fear? It's helpful to understand it if you are to make peace with it. Generally, when humans experience fear we feel agitation, anxiety, apprehension, dread, or even terror. These feelings are caused by our perception of the presence or nearness of danger, pain, loss, embarrassment, or humiliation. Often what we fear is not the event itself, but the unknown outcome.

A wise soul once told me, "Events of your day—meetings, presentations, conflicts, and so on—may seem difficult or may not go

Chapter 14: Mind and Thoughts

your way, but you need to see them for what they are—*transactions*. You may not want to go through the hassle or experience the anxiety, but tomorrow you will see this was a mere transaction, not a big deal." Though fleeting and momentary, our conditioning makes us view these transactions as so important that they allow our anxiety about them to grow out of control. Any time I'm not looking forward to a meeting or encounter, I remember this advice. Immediately, the temporary nature of the encounter is put into proper perspective.

Fear lowers your vibrational frequency. Aside from feeling immensely unpleasant, fear is pure static—dense, low-vibrating energy that blocks your frequency. There are many ways to shift your perspective about fear, allowing your vibrational frequency to clear and heighten. What if each time you experience fear, you shift your mindset to one of curiosity and exploration—more of a "what if" approach? Let the powerful emotions associated with fear dissipate and allow curiosity, faith, and learning to take over. It can be helpful when you find yourself experiencing fear to focus on your breathing and your Sacred Sevens. This will help you to retain your center and your perspective.

Another extremely effective means for shifting away from fear is to turn to gratitude, the nemesis of fear. Despite the circumstance or event causing the fear, take a moment to express gratitude for all that you have in this life. Give thanks for the courage and audacity you have been given to step outside of your comfort zone. You may still feel uncomfortable, but when you face your fears head-on, your confidence begins to grow. Look at fear as a bridge to the new you. Once you cross over, you'll have added immeasurably to your coping bag of tricks, and will feel expanded.

Where courage prevails and fear subsides, you heighten your energetic vibrations and clear a space for inspiration and creativity to speak to you. You cannot begin to fathom your possibilities—but the universe sees your limitless potentiality in ways you have never imagined. Your resolve, driven by your soul's purpose, carries more power and potential than any anxiety brought on by a transaction. As you summon the strength to move through fear, you will be guided by your internal instruction system and other signs, signals, symbols, and synchronicities.

One last note—it is essential that through awareness and listening to your feelings you develop the ability to discern between doubt and fear. Listen to doubt. When doubt enters your mind, stop. If possible, still yourself or meditate before moving forward. When doubt is present, you must clear your mind and go to your state of motionlessness and tranquility to look for an answer before taking action. Doubt may be your internal instruction system guiding you in another direction.

Courage

Courage is an essential aspect of the Living with Certainty philosophy, and goes hand in hand with faith. It's a state of mind and spirit that provides you with the moral strength to persevere—the "anti-fear," if you will. A full life will routinely put you in situations that force you out of your comfort zone. This is what you want—a life that pushes, challenges, and forces you to grow and expand, not one that shelters you from forward movement. Each time you show courage, you demonstrate your commitment to a goal or purpose that you have deemed to be more significant than your fear.

Having the courage to take risks and try new things opens your life to possibilities of which you may have never conceived. You can't bring positive and lasting change to your life without being open to risk. You must be willing to stretch yourself to see how far you can go and what you are capable of. Be brave and bold. You can't allow fear of the unknown or a previous pattern of not taking risks to keep you from trying new things.

It's worth walking through fear just to experience how good bravery and courage feel on the other side. This is an example of that fine give-and-take relationship between mind and body that's essential for continued personal growth. Your mind prepares the body to move through an event. Despite any fear, anxiety, or mental obstacles your mind creates, the body is fully capable of undertaking whatever action becomes necessary. At the same time, your mind also rises to the occasion. Before you know it, the event is over and your mind not only dissolves the fear, but it also wants to celebrate—"I am brave! Let's do it again!"

Confidence
Confidence is the realization that you can believe in your own powers and abilities. Confidence is essential for achievement because it relates directly to your own self-respect. Your confidence will grow as you experience small wins that prepare you to take on bigger challenges. Each time you take soul-view–aligned action, you build confidence and self-esteem.

Strive to maintain a positive mental attitude and proactive approach to life. Stand tall and hold your head high. This is the stance of confident, successful people, and helps to create a self-perception that you are, in fact, confident. It's important, however, not to confuse confidence with ego or conceit. True confidence stems from respecting the value of all human life, embracing your purposeful authenticity, and not being easily swayed or angered by others' opinions. Remember, on this very day, even as you sit reading this book, you have untapped, limitless, one-of-a-kind potential that can make the world a better place. Know your strengths and leverage them. Be proud of all that makes you unique. Make yourself visible. Position yourself strategically.

19. Affirmations

*"It's the repetition of affirmations that leads to belief.
And once that belief becomes a deep conviction,
things begin to happen."*
—Claude M. Bristol

An affirmation is an emphatic, positive statement declared to be true. Scientists have identified certain areas of the brain, such as the reticular activating system (RAS), which functions in concert with the visual parts of our brain to focus our conscious attention on subjects and notions that will help us to reach our goals, while filtering out those things that are extraneous. The RAS is triggered by encoding or programming goals into our subconscious mind, the powerful apparatus that reacts to affirmations, visualization, and goal-setting—all of which are increasingly being accepted as valid, scientific means for self-improvement.[11]

Marianne Williamson said, "Our deepest fear is not that we are inadequate. Our deepest fear is that we are powerful beyond measure. It is our light, not our darkness that most frightens us. We ask ourselves, who am I to be brilliant, gorgeous, talented, fabulous? Actually, who are you not to be? You are a child of God. Your playing small does not serve the world. There is nothing enlightened about shrinking so that other people won't feel insecure around you. We are all meant to shine, as children do. We were born to make manifest the glory of God that is within us. It's not just in some of us; it's in everyone. And as we let our own light shine, we unconsciously give other people permission to do the same. As we are liberated from our own fear, our presence automatically liberates others."[12]

If they are to have any merit, affirmations must be powered by feeling, belief, and emotion, as if they have already manifested in reality. You are attempting to reprogram or trick your subconscious mind into thinking that you have already achieved what you want. Repeating affirmations on a daily basis has a powerful effect on shaping you, your self-perception, and your life. Give yourself permission to be amazing.

Remember, all of your affirmations must be aligned with your inspired soul-view if you are to be able to have an impact on and align with Source energy. The words only matter to the extent that they stir up the emotion that leads to the feelings—the feelings are what matter because their vibrations have a direct affect on the powerful unseen from which our lives are made manifest.

How do you start? Each morning, begin with an affirmation repeated over and over again. Close your eyes. Take a deep breath. Clear your mind. Begin very simply by exhaling and thinking the words, "I love myself." This alone is powerful. Repetition is important. You must repeat your affirmations with conviction so that at your core you believe what you are saying. Make sure that any words or thoughts that cross your mind are positive. Focus on just a few affirmations that go to the heart of what you are trying to achieve.

Keep a journal page devoted solely to positive affirmations, and write them repeatedly every day. If you really want to make a significant change in your thought patterns, read them several times throughout the day over a period of months, and say them out loud while looking at yourself in the mirror.

Try this powerful Living with Certainty affirmation: "I am one with Source energy and, therefore, I am connected with every other aspect of the universe. I live in alignment with my inspired soul-view and purposeful authenticity, allowing myself to be the powerful, compassionate, fulfilled, healthy, and loving co-creator of my deep-soul joy-filled life."

20. Kindness and Tolerance
"My religion is very simple. My religion is kindness."
—His Holiness The Dalai Lama

Kindness combines numerous individual Energy Enablers, such as universal interconnectivity, compassion, acceptance, and forgiveness into a single general approach to your thoughts and daily life. As you live with certainty, you'll find that most of the Energy Enablers begin to come quite naturally to you, and become second nature; one leads to another.

If you are to be kind, you must also be tolerant. This means you recognize differences and still respect them. You allow others to exist in their own beliefs without interfering, hindering, or quelling them in any way. Mastering tolerance in Earthly physicality is one of the most difficult of human challenges. Tolerance naturally ensues from living with certainty. Just imagine the kind of universe we could create and experience if we all projected kinder, gentler, more tolerant energy out into the web of universal interconnectivity.

You won't be able to extend kindness and compassion to others if you don't feel worthy of it yourself. The energy you project toward yourself is the very energy that you project out to the universe. If you treat yourself with a lack of love and respect, you are not only creating static for yourself, but will also treat others with that same lack of love and respect. You will not be able to view the world through a kind, compassionate lens until you first view and treat yourself in this way. The quickest way to change how you feel is to extend your love or a hand to someone else in need. Expressing loving feelings toward others—even toward animals—is proven to be good for your health, and is certainly good for your psyche.

You have much to give; offer it up to the world every day in all of your interactions. Each day, commit as many acts of kindness as you possibly can. This is how you get others to pay it forward. At the same time, notice and give thanks for every act of kindness bestowed upon you. Wish nothing but the best for others, and view everyone through a non-judgmental lens of compassion and truth.

21. Optimism

"No pessimist ever discovered the secret of the stars, or sailed to an uncharted land, or opened a new heaven to the human spirit."
—Helen Keller

Your attitude represents your energy, which is either positive or negative. How you view the events of your life is your choice. But remember this—your emotions are inextricably linked to your attitude. In order to create and maintain high-frequency vibrations, it's crucial that you remain aware of, and constantly adjust, your attitude. Living with certainty means you are living from a positive, soul-based state, and are maintaining a consistently faith-driven, upbeat, optimistic attitude. This approach is intended to keep your mind, body, and spirit at an optimal level of vibrational frequency.

Living with certainty causes you to look for the significance and meaning in every moment. Eventually, as this becomes core to how you approach life, you'll frequently ask yourself, *What is this moment or experience here to teach me?* This isn't to say that you turn a blind eye to negative events, or deny that they are taking place. It means, however, that you live with perspective and keep your eye on teaching moments.

Living with optimism has mental, physical, and spiritual benefits. Research has provided hard evidence that optimism positively affects our health, including a lower risk of heart attack, a healthier immune system, the ability to better cope with pain and life-threatening illnesses, quicker recovery times, and a general belief that we will get healthier. Optimists tend to believe that a negative event was a fluke and may likely never happen again. The future looks bright to optimists because they expect good things to happen.

Optimism keeps your energy vibrating at a high-frequency level. The choice you must make every day is whether to see the glass as half empty or as half full. The power to change your life is in your mind and imagination. Once you see and believe in a better life for yourself, you are unstoppable.

If you're not naturally hardwired to be optimistic, you can alter your disposition toward pessimism through awareness of your thought patterns. This may require working with a therapist. Anytime a negative thought enters your mind, you must challenge it by flipping a switch to a more positive thought.

Negativity

How do you stay positive in the face of negativity, particularly when surrounded by negative people with whom you cannot or do not want to sever relations? This is one of the biggest challenges you will face as you live with certainty. You have to take action to change the subject, change the focus, bring a more positive perspective, or just come right out and ask the person to stop being so negative.

Rather than worry about offending someone, you must think in positive terms. You are doing everyone involved a favor when you change the energy from negative to positive. Most negative people need all the help they can get. Whenever possible, choose only to maintain close relationships with people who are positive.

22. The Law of Attraction

"I am no longer cursed by poverty because I took possession of my own mind, and that mind has yielded me every material thing I want, and much more than I need. But this power of mind is a universal one, available to the humblest person as it is to the greatest."
—Andrew Carnegie

Co-creation is the ability to see in your mind's eye that which you want to be and experience in your life, before it actually manifests itself in Earthly physicality. This visualization technique allows you to transform moments of your life into authentic soul-view–aligned feelings. These become magnets of opportunity for Source energy to reflect the content of these feelings back to you. This is part of the Law of Attraction process. You are encoding and instructing universal intelligence on how to act, to the extent that you can through your power as co-creator. This effort provides the internal blueprint for the powerful unseen to act upon.

Your thoughts are powerful points of attraction—vibrations that emanate out into the universe, pulling to you those things on which you focus. Your sustained and repetitive thoughts carry the power to vibrate messages to Source energy. However, whether you are successful at co-creating your life through your thoughts depends upon whether you are aligned with your inspired soul-view. This, in turn, determines whether you are in alignment with the energy flow of the universe and your spiritual power frequency. The quality of the energy you put out creates the experience you will receive in return.

So, what does it mean to co-create your life? Quite simply, it's the process through which you participate, to the extent that you can, in the creation of the life the universe always intended for you to live. Source energy dreams bigger and with more abundance than we can even begin to fathom. It has intelligence and insight that we cannot comprehend. We must, then, serenely accept that we are enveloped in a connected, yielding, and bending world that allows us to participate in the creation of our lives.

What can you control throughout your Earthly journey? You can control your awareness of every moment, and whether you live a life of purposeful authenticity and deep-soul joy. You can control your thoughts, feelings, and beliefs. You can control whether you see and receive guidance from signs, symbols, signals, and synchronicities; and whether you live in tune with your internal instruction system. You can control whether you are moving your life forward through inspired soul-view–aligned action.

Does the all-powerful creative energy field respond to negative, non-soul-view–aligned thoughts, emotions, and beliefs? You bet it does. As you focus on what you don't want, your energy becomes dense and low-vibrating—and this energy appears to attract dense, low-vibrating events and circumstances while removing you from the flow of your spiritual power frequency.

Thankfully, positive thoughts carry immensely powerful energy that affects you to your core. Positive thoughts can only be made manifest when they are aligned with your inspired soul-view and purposeful authenticity. Simply thinking about what would be nice to have in your life will not attract these things unless they are somehow aligned with your inspired soul-view. Otherwise, we would all just wish everything we want into existence. Further, enough time has passed since the concept of The Law of Attraction exploded into mainstream society that we've all had ample time to try it and see that it alone does not make manifest our wishes.

Kristi's Power Enabler

We have a conscious choice to make as we face the ups and downs of every day life. We can either fall apart and make matters worse than they really are through our undisciplined thought, or we can use our Source energy-gifted faculties to help us to remain as strong and steady as possible by controlling our thoughts in such a way that they serve to move us out of the darkness and into the light. As you feel negativity growing within you, the only answer is to choose to think differently, more positively. You can do this.

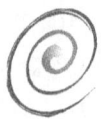

CHAPTER 15

Actions

"Put your heart, mind and soul into even your smallest acts. That is the secret to success."
—Swami Sivananda

KNOWLEDGE DOESN'T DIRECTLY TRANSLATE to enlightenment, or lead to change. As humans, we need to employ action in order to realize any level of accomplishment or success in life. Our physical beings are designed to constantly reach, endeavor, strive, and explore.

You have to be present and fully participate in your life. This means rolling up your sleeves and doing the required work in order to move forward. While the universe works on your behalf, you—as co-creator—must also do your share. We've all heard the phrase "Carpe diem—Seize the Day." We can do this most effectively by taking inspired soul-view–aligned action. In this way, lasting change becomes possible. Your intention to undertake the journey toward an authentic spiritual life is an essential and powerful beginning. But you must also have a plan or strategy in place.

What is the difference between action and inspired soul-view–aligned action? Mere action can include the monotonous activities of your day-to-day duties and tasks, which in no way move your spiritual life forward. Most of us live some aspects of our lives logically identifying our goals, and knowing what we must do next. This is the linear, predictable route to accomplishment that includes focusing on fulfilling tasks, and being conscientious and disciplined. However, inspired soul-view–aligned action is less obvious. It drives and supplements your linear, logical actions by causing you to feel instinctually compelled to do things that may not seem logical at all. Your inspired soul-view–aligned action will be revealed to you through your internal instruction system. Source energy is guiding you as you act with purpose and authenticity.

As your mind experiences authentic action and progress, you create conditions for your energy to vibrate at optimal levels. When you reach a point where you are consistently satisfied and proud of your soul-view–aligned actions, the most succinct reflection of who you are, you won't want to live any other way.

23. Risk and Leaps of Faith

*"We can easily forgive a child who is afraid of the dark;
the real tragedy of life is when adults are afraid of the light."*
—Plato

Great accomplishment takes contemplation, effort—and usually some risk. Since we'll never have all of the answers about how our mysterious universe works, our greatest certainty in life is to move forward according to how we feel. To do this, we must to some extent be willing to take a leap of faith. Certainly, the risks we choose to take should involve enough analysis and planning to help ensure success. It has been said that guts without calculation is foolish. However, as you live with certainty, what may have previously seemed like risk can now be viewed as inspired soul-view–aligned action.

Living with certainty requires that you have the courage to trust your instincts and vision, and have faith that they hold great things for you. When something deeply resonates with you, it is guidance to which you should listen. Welcome the unknown when your internal instruction system is speaking to you. Instinct-aligned risk holds the promise of possibility. Let this inspire you, and infuse you with courage and faith.

When you take a risk or a leap of faith that feels aligned with your inspired soul-view, you are honoring your intuition and your connection to Source energy. If it feels right, if your internal instruction system is saying *yes, yes, yes,* what's wrong with a little adventure?

Wouldn't you prefer to take an instinct-driven risk than to spend the rest of your days wondering, *What if?* When you have a deep-seated confidence that you're moving forward in alignment with your inspired soul-view, you are co-creating the life the universe always intended for you to live. This is Living with Certainty.

Risk contains an element of paradox—if you don't take an instinct-driven, calculated chance, you'll feel as if you've let yourself down. One part of you may be ready and raring to go, while another hesitates. When you allow these opportunities to pass by, you remove yourself from universal flow and your spiritual power frequency, and choose not to co-create the life the universe always intended for you to live. Be bold and have faith. Your internal instruction system won't lead you astray.

24. Effort and Excellence

"To win in this life, you simply have to give your all, every bit of yourself ... . Life cannot deny itself to the person who gives everything."
—Norman Vincent Peale

To live with certainty, excellence needs to become a habit. Everything you undertake should be given your fullest effort. Hard work, self-discipline, awareness, and commitment—essentially giving your all—are required. When you bring your full effort to bear as you undertake soul-view–aligned action, you are capable of creating exceptional merit and virtue. You also align with the flow of your spiritual power frequency, which works with you to move you even more quickly toward the life the universe always intended for you to live.

To be present and give your all at every moment requires conscious effort. This isn't about performing well for your boss, or using smoke and mirrors to create the illusion of high performance. You do this for yourself—no one but you will know if you truly are giving 100 percent. You need to experience the satisfaction of doing your best.

It's through applying yourself fully to your endeavors that development and growth happen. One day you're flipping burgers to the very best of your ability. Before you know it, you're managing the restaurant, then multiple restaurants. Next, you're running the company. Joyous winners in life aren't satisfied with the status quo. They crave self-exploration and development, and drive themselves to new heights every day.

Your work environment can provide the ideal place to hone your unique capabilities, and to test what you really enjoy doing. While you may know that your current job isn't in alignment with your purposeful authenticity, accept the reality of where you are today while firmly visualizing where you are headed. Although some days you may feel as though you're merely punching a clock, approaching your time on the job with a mindset of excellence will allow you to make significant contributions, while also developing and learning about yourself.

Apply yourself, rise to the occasion, be present, and give your all. It matters. Have faith that the universe will provide you with the right contacts and opportunities at the right time, usually when you're least expecting it.

25. Commitment, Persistence, and Perseverance

"Fall seven times, stand up eight."
—Japanese Proverb

To fully participate in the co-creation of your life, you must be infused with an inquisitive nature and the authentic desire to explore your life—pushing here, challenging there, and always seeking new paths and options. To truly surpass old limits and boundaries, you must constantly stretch beyond your comfort zone.

Perseverance is a quality that can serve you well throughout life—and it's an important aspect of Living with Certainty. Throughout your journey, Source energy will be relentless in communicating guidance to you. Live your life with the same sense of persistence with which Source energy attempts to guide you.

Some of us have more to overcome than others. Illness, disability, and geographic limitations are just a few of the many disadvantages that some people consider to be insurmountable odds. However, we can all cite numerous examples of people who have overcome great challenges to lead purposeful lives of deep-soul joy. Building something of value that will endure requires a complete absence of a victim mentality, along with aptitude, skill, commitment, reasonableness, wisdom, and resolve.

We live in a chaotic, unpredictable world. You may be one of the most gifted people on the planet, but without a vision, focus, and commitment, it's unlikely that you will ever achieve any level of greatness or success. On the other hand, a person of average intellect and talent can set the world on fire with determination. Staying focused, even in the face of great odds and uncertainty, will ultimately make the various obstacles you encounter seem less daunting.

Determination involves faith and trust that every setback provides an opportunity for you to awaken and learn. The most successful individuals have the resilience and pluckiness to pick themselves up after disappointment, learn the lesson, and then carry on. You must expect that as you begin to live with certainty and in alignment with your purposeful authenticity that life will continue to affect you with its inevitable ups and downs. One day's revolution or breakthrough will be followed by another day's collapse. Through living with certainty, you will learn to use each and every one of these experiences as an opportunity to awaken.

Experts say that it takes twenty-one days to break a habit. It will take longer than that to incorporate the Living with Certainty tenets and Energy Enablers into your life. If you initially do nothing more than try to feel good by following your gut feelings and emotions, you're doing enough to set the foundation for the rest of your efforts. You're going to be living with a new toolkit, and it takes time to learn to use these tools proficiently. Commitment and consistency will be needed to get you through the first weeks of this new approach to life.

Living with Certainty doesn't guarantee that you'll always be filled with joy, or that you will never again experience pain. That's not realistic. It will, however, encourage you not to give up on yourself. To abandon this powerful, mysterious, magical journey would be to deny yourself the life the universe always intended for you to live.

26. Change

"They must often change, who would be constant in happiness or wisdom."
—Confucius

Any time you make a change, you transform yourself as you pass from one stage to another. It is a waste of your time and effort to try to avoid or circumvent change. Your very choices create change—and that's a good thing.

Just making the decision to change is a big and necessary part of integrating acceptance of change into your life. Living with Certainty is about taking small, achievable steps forward all throughout your day. Don't expect flawlessness or perfection. Just improvements. Strive for actions that are as aligned with your inspired soul-view as possible. Over time, this will become a more natural approach to your life. The key is to be consistent.

The perceived loss of security, along with a fear of the unknown and the unfamiliar, can scare us and cause anxiety. This is because we often place too much emphasis on what we are losing, rather than on what we stand to gain. You needn't fear, however, that your life will change instantaneously. What you do leading up to the change—to prepare for it—takes time, and will allow you the space to wrap your mind around the fact that better things are on the horizon. Making choices that are aligned with your inspired soul-view will feel good, comforting, and secure; it's the change you've longed for.

Change is a fact of human life, of Earthly physicality. Any time you make a long-overdue change, you free blocked energy and clear the way to reengage in the flow of your spiritual power frequency. Don't let the only time you open yourself to change be when you experience a major blow that forces you out of your old habits and patterns.

When you resist needed change, you disengage from flow and create heavy, stagnant energy. Remaining stuck in your ways and avoiding change doesn't allow for growth and enlightenment. As difficult as you may find it to remain centered and calm during these times, just remember that your essence isn't altered just because things around you are changing. Your soul-center remains steady, even as your ego-personality reacts emotionally to life's inescapable ups and downs.

27. Learning

"Learning is not attained by chance, it must be sought for with ardor and attended to with diligence."
—Abigail Adams

Continual, life-long learning is essential for being an insightful, joyous, and fulfilled person. Personal development enables you to experience more joy. Learning requires awareness, an astute nature, and curiosity about every aspect of life. You must be open to lessons that come your way, and acknowledge that you don't have all of the answers. When you approach your daily life with the mindset that every moment intentionally exists as a personal learning experience, much of the anxiety you feel about the future will begin to fade away.

Living with Certainty requires a willingness to grow beyond all that you know. When you are safe, stable, and secure in the fundamentals of your life, it's easy to stay put. But if you allow yourself to settle on this path, you'll never fully explore your personal potential.

Source energy knows where you are developmentally at any point in time. Your internal compass is constantly being tested and developed in new, expansive ways. If you need certain knowledge in order to make the right choice in a future circumstance, rest assured you'll be presented with challenges and opportunities to advance your learning that will prepare you.

Very often, the lessons that you need to learn aren't the ones you would expect. Your greatest problem may ultimately be your greatest treasure, ultimately providing the "aha" lesson from which abundance will emanate. The next time you hit a rough patch, ask yourself, *What is this intended to teach me?* Embrace the fact that it's this unwelcome, unwanted stuff that feels so harsh that ultimately brings the lessons that allow you to develop the insight and knowledge to ascend to the next level.

In every moment, every encounter, and every circumstance of our daily lives, we encounter teachers. At the same time, we are given opportunities to be the teacher—to listen, show compassion, and serve as a light for someone in need. Often, it's the most problematic and difficult people who teach us the most. It's the same for some of the most negative relationships in our lives—they were put there for us to learn from, and to prompt us to take a closer look at ourselves.

Interestingly, the extent to which we learn from past experiences varies greatly between individuals. Researchers from the Max Planck Institutes for Human Cognitive and Brain Science and Neurological Research, as well as the University of Giessen and University of Bonn in Germany, are studying the gene characteristics associated with addictive and compulsive behaviors and how they may result in "some insensitivity to negative consequences of self-destructive behaviors. This might be linked to a general deficit in learning from errors."[13] While some of us may not be able to learn from our experiences to the same extent as others, adopting the perspective that curve balls are learning opportunities can be an effective coping strategy.

The world will never stop changing. If you cease to grow, you'll only become frustrated as the world around you continues to transform. A willingness to learn and adapt, along with cultivating the ability to alter your habits and expectations, will allow you to feel more joy and satisfaction in all facets of your life.

28. Deceleration and Balance

*"If you're moving all the time,
you're not stopping to be or think or experience nature."*
—Maria Shriver

Living with certainty demands that you create balance in your life—inside and outside. Balance doesn't mean all things in equal portions; it's about giving the most energy to what is the most important. It's about the ability to remain on your feet, as it were, when the waves crash against you. Once you achieve this state, you can begin to sort through your feelings and thoughts from the perspective of your internal instruction system. Consistent meditation can be just the ticket for advancing your mental and emotional processes to a higher and more balanced level.

A life of balance may not sound particularly exciting or stimulating. But a balanced life is hardly a boring life. You simply can't move through life without the occasional pause. While some aspects of life require a go-go-go approach, some of your biggest mistakes can come from taking action that was lacking in good judgment or completely out of alignment with your internal instruction system. We can find more balance, simplicity, and peace in our lives by pausing.

Staying balanced can take some getting used to. You may feel that your life is chaotic and hectic, and that you have no time, focus, or inclination to level out and find your center. When you move blindly through life this way, you live without awareness of the here and now, and without consulting your inspired soul-view or internal instruction system. The pressure to accumulate more, or have the best house, car, and jewelry can leave you feeling that you have no choice but to move at a breakneck pace to hold things together. This need for speed becomes a pattern, and you allow life's pleasures and real purpose to pass you by.

If your calendar is overwhelmed with tasks and activities that are not at all in alignment with your purposeful authenticity, it's time to assess what needs to go. If you're being carried along by the flow of your Outlook calendar instead of your spiritual power frequency, you're in trouble. Your bank account may be in great shape, but how is your spiritual account measuring up?

Many people try to stay busy as much as possible to avoid dealing with their feelings, or with problems that don't have easy solutions. Others have difficulty slowing down because they're uncomfortable just *being*.

Moving through life at a breakneck pace is wasted time because you leave no room for spiritual enlightenment or meaning to enter and help guide you. You must slow down if you are to awaken to receive Spirit in your life. You'll still have plenty of time to enjoy a full life of purposeful activity, hobbies, family, friends, exercise, love, and anything else you value. You'll accomplish all you want far more effectively when you approach it from a centered, balanced, and relaxed state.

Source energy has its own tempo and flow. Find time to spend in stillness and silence, even if it means stopping at a park to sit down at a picnic table for a few minutes on your way home from work, just to enjoy the silence. By doing this, you'll change the quality and texture of your life.

You must slow down to become aware of your subtle thoughts, feelings, and instincts. You're less likely to make poor choices and costly errors when you decelerate. Any task will be better completed from a place of balance, control, and calm.

29. Simplicity

"There is no greatness where there is not simplicity, goodness, and truth."
—Leo Nikolaevich Tolstoy

To be simple is to be without attachment, vanity, or deceit. Simplicity weakens your need for attachment. With simplicity, you create room—essential white space—for peace and contentment to enter your life. You need to create this white space both internally and externally in order to live with certainty. As you become internally fulfilled, you require far less externally in order to experience joy.

As our society has grown more chaotic and materialistic, we seem to have rejected the premise that a simple life can be a joyous life. But simplifying your life is a huge step forward toward reconciling your inner and outer selves. As you clear space, you announce to Source energy your readiness to pursue a spiritual life. Living simply is living clean and clear—your heart, mind, thoughts, beliefs, and energy become open, receptive, and as closely aligned with Source energy as possible.

For your mind and energy to be optimally focused and clear, it's necessary to eliminate (or lessen the focus on) aspects of your life that add to your anxiety and stress. If you have real or metaphorical closets filled with junk, you'll experience static that will prevent you from vibrating energy at the purest, highest frequency possible. Deliberate orderliness and focus need to be your goal in every major area of your life—mind, body, spirit, and environment. As you cleanse your outer life, you create internal space. If you can't completely eliminate certain things from your environment or experience, explore ways to lessen their impact on your daily life.

Once you simplify, give thanks for this space and acknowledge how good the energy feels. As you de-clutter, you physically experience a relief that's tantamount to exhaling. It feels as if a weight has been lifted. This is actually the clearing of your energy as you align more closely with that which is pure and high-vibrating.

30. Goal-Setting and Planning

"Our goals can only be reached through a vehicle of a plan, in which we must fervently believe, and upon which we must vigorously act. There is no other route to success."
—Vincent van Gogh

Planning and goal-setting are fundamental aspects of keeping yourself moving forward toward a life of joy and purposeful authenticity, and aid in the achievement of your desires and success. After you've discovered your inspired soul-view, you must set your goals and devise an action plan. You should have both personal and professional goals that provide direction and give you something to visualize. What habits and skills do you need? What needs to be changed or thought of differently? What pitfalls are lurking that can take you off track and stymie your progress? Don't leave things to chance—be strategic and plan.

Goal-setting and planning are different, however, from attempting to control every aspect of your life. Remember, openness and flexibility are essential if you are to live in alignment with the flow of your spiritual power frequency. You can't control the flow. The only thing you should try to control is your ability to maintain a high personal vibrational frequency.

Fundamental to Living with Certainty is accepting that you don't know everything, nor do you have the power to control this vast, magnificent universe. Since you don't know everything, there's no possible way for you to know what's right for others. If control is a problem for you, find a couple of opportunities to let something go, to allow someone else to take charge, to see how it feels not to attempt to manage every aspect of your life. Practice the freedom that comes from releasing your grip.

31. Responsibility

"The willingness to accept responsibility for one's own life is the source from which self-respect springs."
—Joan Didion

Responsibility means you are answerable to someone or something, and are morally, legally, or ethically accountable and bound by duty or obligation. When you are responsible, you are dependable. To live with certainty is to be responsible for your own conduct. You must honor your word, be reliable, and follow through on commitments to others and to yourself. Others must be able to count on you in both word and deed. Responsibility keeps you moving forward with integrity.

As you accept responsibility for your life, you begin to take your choices and decisions much more seriously, and to consistently see things through to completion. This requires that you no longer lay blame on others. Avoiding responsibility leaves you in a negative, low-energy place. As you learn to live in alignment with your purposeful authenticity and internal instruction system, you will more naturally want to take the reigns of your life with full accountability.

32. Well-Being

"The concept of total wellness recognizes that our every thought, word, and behavior affects our greater health and well-being. And we, in turn, are affected not only emotionally but also physically and spiritually."
—Greg Anderson

Optimal well-being is the balanced, nourishing, and vital assimilation between your body, mind, emotions, spirit, and physical environment. When we are out of balance in any one of these areas, we experience unrest and discomfort and are unable to vibrate energy at a fine, pure frequency level. Feeling vital and energized are essential aspects of joy. As you live with certainty, you will naturally want to become healthier and more balanced, and to take better care of your physical body.

Our health is a fusion of every aspect of how we have been living our life—power frequency, nutrition, movement, thoughts, beliefs, emotional states, karma, choices, and actions. Maintaining optimal balance and peak physical energy levels takes some level of discipline, but it needn't be at the expense of pleasure and joy. Ridding yourself of bad health habits, such as eating bad foods, not exercising, exceeding your healthiest weight, abusing drugs, or indulging in too much alcohol or tobacco, will ultimately allow you to find your balance and feel much better. Once you discover what feels really good to you, you'll naturally gravitate to that state and become motivated to do what it takes to feel that way. With vitality, peace, and joy in your mind and body, you feel better and your problems seem manageable.

How you care for and feed yourself physically, mentally, and spiritually is a sign of self-respect, and affects the quality of your energy vibrations. Your emotional state is directly connected to how much sleep you've had, how you're eating, how frequently you meditate, and how much you're exercising.

Your Body as Temple

American culture and poor early conditioning have caused many people to not love their bodies. Consistent negative and toxic thoughts throw us out of balance, and create an internal environment that is conducive to illness and disease.

This is unfortunate because our bodies were created by the universe to serve as our soul's house, a wondrous and sacred part of nature that should be revered. For this reason, you should approach your body as a sacred temple that deserves to be cared for and nurtured.

This doesn't mean superficial admiration for your body, but rather a deep respect for the heart that pumps your blood, the eyes that give you sight, the ears that provide you with sound, and the bones and muscles that give you strength.

Your Health and Living with Certainty

Research studies funded by the John Templeton Foundation, and published in leading medical journals, have shown that spirituality has measurable health benefits, including increased life expectancy. While spirituality and religion have been shown to be good for our health, these studies don't indicate what it is about religion and spirituality that provides these benefits. More than half of America's 125 medical schools now offer courses on spirituality and health, up from just three in 1992.[14]

Studies likewise reveal that there seems to be a direct connection between your mental state and physical health—negative begets negative, and positive begets positive. Ironically, the kinder you are to yourself and the more love you extend to yourself, the more likely you are to treat your body in ways that make it healthier.

Nutrition, Moderation, and Weight Loss

With wisdom comes the inherent appreciation for living with moderation and self-restraint. You must become more practical, and develop inner discipline. Your choices usually carry great consequence (whether you always realize it or not), and excess rarely serves you well. When it comes to weight loss, it's essential that you stay in the moment and not continually look into the future as a long, daunting, deprivation-filled journey. Instead, focus on making the best choices in the moment about how you eat and exercise. The journey takes care of itself as you put together moment after moment of good choices.

Actress and health and wellness activist Mariel Hemingway said, "Making different choices in eating is something we need to look at as part of our spiritual journey. It is more than food ... eating is ritual and food is the most pure form of energy. If you think of food as a spiritual energy source that is not only feeding your body but your soul then you have a different resonance with food and food becomes your healing, your joy, and your pleasure instead of a way that you anesthetize yourself and run away from your feelings or beat yourself up."[15]

Everything you ingest has the ability to heal or hinder your health. Eventually, the detrimental effects of poor food choices take their toll on your body, your energy, and your ability to be a spouse, parent, friend, and co-worker. Your lifestyle must be one that allows you to be and feel energetic, healthy, and vibrant. Good health is an essential part of your being. When you feel healthy, you radiate it to others.

33. Karma

"Karma is the eternal assertion of human freedom .... Our thoughts, our words, and deeds are the threads of the net which we throw around ourselves."
—Swami Vivekananda

Many of us know karma as the law of cause and effect. In Hinduism and Buddhism, karma refers to the principle that our actions and conduct during the successive phases of our existence determine our future in this life or in other incarnations. It's easiest to understand karma as the consequences that follow our actions.

Karma has nothing to do with morality, but has everything to do with energy. It serves to make us more responsible and thoughtful regarding our thoughts and actions, all of which are comprised of energy. When our energy is imbalanced and negative, there will be a reaction. There are no haphazard, chance occurrences. Rather, as the saying goes, what goes around comes around.

According to karma, the state of your life is exactly as it is right now because of every thought, action, and belief that you have had throughout your life. As you vibrate energy optimally through living with certainty, your karma is pure, good, and in alignment with Source energy. If you're acting recklessly and selfishly, rest assured that you'll eventually suffer painful repercussions and consequences that are in proportion to your actions. You really cannot get away with anything; eventually, you will live through the consequences of your transgressions. The law of karma should make you more careful and responsible about your choices.

Your karma has everything to do with your intentions. Nothing that you do at someone else's expense will have an energetically good outcome. When you deliberately inflict harm or abuse, you create significant negative energy for which you will experience a karmic backlash. If you want goodness in your life, be responsible for bringing more goodness into the world.

With karma, you're continually receiving or being presented with lessons required for your continued development and enlightenment. If you act in ways that are less than enlightened, the universe will present you with opportunities to learn poignant lessons that help you to heal and move forward. Karma ensures that you continually receive the necessary lessons and teachings, whether you like them or not. This is the prescription for attaining enlightenment—a steady diet of learning opportunities intended to heal and strengthen your soft spots. You cannot create negative energy and problems for others and still expect to experience happiness and peace for yourself. Karma won't allow it.

34. Using Luck
*"I am a great believer in luck,
and I find the harder I work, the more I have of it."*
—Thomas Jefferson

Oprah Winfrey often echoes Earl Nightingale when she says that there's no such thing as luck; there is only preparation meeting the moment of opportunity.[16] What is luck but a favorable outcome? Lucky people have the guts to take advantage of the opportunities that surround all of us. Unfortunately, we aren't all good at recognizing these opportunities.

Your own actions and thoughts are most often what create your luck. You must always put forth your best effort, prepare adequately, and take soul-view–aligned action. Typically, it's when you lack true belief in yourself and your abilities that you miss lucky opportunities. Once you align with your inspired soul-view and begin working in the right direction, luck will intervene every time that goodness is extended out into the world. Don't ever give up on luck, or say that you have bad luck. As long as you continue to take soul-view–aligned action, luck will never give up on you.

35. Journals and Writing

"The value of writing our thoughts and feelings lies in reducing inhibition and organizing our complicated mental and emotional lives."
—James W. Pennebaker, Ph.D.

Communication is an innate human need, and journaling serves this need while also functioning as a cleansing practice. It clears your mind and creates space for the next wave of thought and inspiration. Journal writing can be extremely cathartic—just getting the words out can provide a tremendous release and allow you to jettison negative thoughts and energies. When you experience an intense emotion, write your feelings, beliefs, and thoughts down. Doing this has the power to relieve stress, which in turn improves physical health through enhanced immune function, and reducing both blood pressure and heart rate.

Keep a journal of your Living with Certainty journey. Document your thoughts, feelings, beliefs, and gratitude, as well as your successes and struggles with the Energy Enablers. When your journal contains heartfelt messages of gratitude, love, and purpose, it provides another connection to Source energy. Put pen to paper about everything you want. As you do this, you are taking the first steps toward bringing what you want into your Earthly experience.

In your journal, record signs, signals, symbols, and synchronous events and what was going on at the time inside and outside of you—your feelings, interpretations of the signs, whether you followed up on hunch or intuition, outcomes, and so on. Also spend time writing about those things that you tend to dwell on—the things that repeatedly come up that cause you to feel any level of negative emotion. By documenting them, you can begin to work through your issues. Waiting until the initial emotion has passed will help you to create distance between yourself and the feelings, enabling you to process them so that you may ultimately learn from them, and then leave them behind.

It's important that you feel safe as you write in your journal, knowing that no one will read or judge the content. Keep your journal in a safe place where no one can find it. If you keep your journal on your computer, make certain that it's password protected, and backed up. If someone reads your journal, it will prevent you from being open and authentic, which is the purpose of journaling in the first place. Feel free to let it all out—no grammatical perfection required.

36. Travel and Exploration
"Travel is fatal to prejudice, bigotry, and narrow-mindedness."
—Mark Twain

Travel is the perfect reinforcing accompaniment to living with certainty. It broadens your perspective, opens you to the joys of new experiences, heightens your senses, and provides exposure to perspectives and world views that you may never have considered before. In many profound ways, travel changes you. It awakens you to the miraculous diversity that exists in our universe in terms of people, nature, terrain, traditions, religion, food, music, and so on.

When you travel to distant places, you'll almost certainly discover new approaches that can be incorporated into your own life. Through your interactions with people in faraway lands, you'll make connections that bring home for you the concept of universal interconnectivity, and experience tremendous gratitude for all that you have. You'll begin to understand how similar we all are, irrespective of where we live, what we believe, or the color of our skin. Our essential humanness will pierce through the veil of differences. You'll gain a sense of your own place in this vast universe. In fact, you needn't travel across oceans to experience different cultures, dialects, food, and customs—in just a day's drive, you can stretch beyond the familiar borders of your hometown and broaden your experience. Any change in perspective does you good.

> ### Kristi's Power Enabler
> *Inspired soul-view–aligned action is the jet fuel that makes Living with Certainty such a mystical, interesting, and joyous journey. This is what co-creation is all about. Contemplative choice that takes into account your driving desires and purpose is an essential aspect of inspired soul-view–aligned action. This requires knowing who you are outside of your ego-personality and allowing your essence to propel your actions. How does your gut feel? What are your emotions telling you? While taking this action may at times require a leap of faith, ultimately it is the most trustworthy action. It feels good and right at your core, and is accompanied by a strong sense of accomplishment, progress, and belief that you are moving in the right direction. It engages you with a sense of certainty that you are moving in alignment with your purpose and potentiality.*

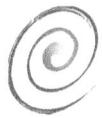

CHAPTER 16

Relationships

"Oh, the comfort—the inexpressible comfort of feeling safe with a person—having neither to weigh thoughts nor measure words ... certain that a faithful hand will take and sift them, keep what is worth keeping, and then with the breath of kindness blow the rest away."
—Dinah Craik

HEALTHY HUMAN BEINGS ARE SOCIAL. We're wired to interact with and relate to others. We require and thrive on love and affection. A good relationship will support and guide you through your life's discovery process. Whether you realize it or not, you are an amalgam of the significant people in your life. The people in our lives change us—and the people with whom you surround yourself can either elevate you or drag you down. As you live with certainty your goal must be to ensure that your relationships consistently lift you up, helping to take you in a positive direction.

You've heard it a hundred times before, but it's *true* that you really must respect and love yourself before you can respect and love others. You simply *can't* have authentic healthy relationships when you don't know and understand yourself. If you don't fundamentally love yourself, your relationships with others will be dysfunctional. You'll be unable to attract fully formed, enlightened individuals into your orbit.

The quality and nature of your relationships and your experiences with people serve as a mirror for you about all aspects of your life, including your level of enlightenment. The things you find irritating in others may well be the very traits that you dislike in yourself. This is why we usually don't get along with the people who are most like us—but the negative feelings we experience about the vices, habits, and behaviors of others often serve to show us an aspect of ourselves that needs healing.

Living with Certainty

Once you're living with certainty, you'll find that your relationships are healthier, and people are attracted to the positive, inspirational, and loving energy you vibrate. When you live with deep-soul joy, you carry it with you everywhere you go. Your life becomes increasingly filled with trusting relationships that enable, encourage, support, and feed higher levels of joy.

As you live with certainty, you can take relationships and their inevitable ups and downs more in stride, accepting and embracing the fact that people move in and out of your life for a purpose. Albeit, you may not realize the purpose these people have served until they are gone from your life. Give thanks for every single person in your life, for they have each taught you something. They have somehow developed or affirmed you.

Your pre-living with certainty relationships may change—or even fall by the wayside—as you begin this journey. Not everyone will appreciate any changes in you if it means that any aspect of your relationship with them is altered. Consciously, they may think they want what's best for you, but subconsciously they may hope your efforts are short-lived and unsuccessful so that their own world isn't affected. They may even discourage you, as they struggle with your decision to live with certainty.

However, healthy relationships allow for and foster your own growth and development, and respect your choices. Those in your inner circle—close family members, friends, and loved ones—may simply want reassurance that you're not going to push them out of your life. Once they understand and believe that this approach will actually make your union with them stronger and more loving, they'll move to your corner. As you explain to others what this Living with Certainty journey is all about, keep in mind that you are not seeking their approval or acceptance.

Spousal Relationship

We spend a great deal of time and effort searching for the so-called perfect mate, but nowhere near that amount of effort nourishing and developing that initial level of passion, romance, and interest. Don't get married if you think that down the road you may be too busy to nourish or care for your relationship. If you are to maintain a strong foundation and remain interested in one another, it's essential that you and your spouse dedicate yourselves to creating time for connection and intimacy, and reminding yourself of the reasons you initially fell in love. Your spouse should be your best friend. The healthiest marriages are characterized by the desire and dedication to help your spouse grow and move forward. You must always remain in your mate's corner—ever dependable and trustworthy. Be a safe haven for one another.

Forming Your Inner Circle

Our closest, loving, most supportive personal relationships—whether family, friends, professionals, support groups, even pets—provide us with powerful encouragement and support that helps to heal us spiritually and physically. The laughter, love, affirmation, support, and kindness extended by your inner circle lifts and strengthens you. As you begin your Living with Certainty journey, you'll develop an inner circle of supporters who will be there when you need them. This inner circle can provide support to you during the toughest times and transitions in your life. Trusted friends or mentors can be the best people to help you break your negative patterns, because they provide support and truth in compassionate and supportive ways. Your inner circle provides a safe place for you to share your blessings, struggles, wisdom, learning, grief, pain, and joy.

As you take stock of your relationships in an effort to determine who is, in fact, a part of your inner circle, consider the following traits an essential threshold: they are grateful for your presence in their lives and cherish their relationship with you as much as you do with them; they have cared about and supported you unconditionally over an extended period of time; you both want to grow together; they bring you joy; they are honorable, ethical, and truthful; they have an optimistic, positive mindset and outlook; they are well-intended; they care about your growth, development, and well-being; you can confide in them and trust them implicitly; they engage in discussions that provide you with essential perspective and focus; and they feed and nurture you, providing a safe place to fall.

Negative Relationships
As you live with certainty, you'll begin every relationship with the intent to be loving and kind. If you find that your kindness isn't reciprocated, or you feel that the relationship's energy exchange is turning dense and negative, do what you can to minimize your exposure to this person—or end the relationship. Red flags should appear when any of the following behaviors rear their ugly heads: egocentricity; stretching the truth or lying; gossip; undependability; lack of integrity; envy or jealousy; flakiness and flightiness; judgment; competition; lack of support; disrespect; or abuse. When a relationship causes you to compromise yourself, your values, and/or your self-respect, it's unhealthy.

Encourage those you love to live with certainty. Give them your full support as you let them know that you do not want them to miss out on the opportunity to live the life the universe always intended for them to live.

37. Family and Teaching the World's Children
*"There are only two lasting bequests we can give our children—
one is roots, the other wings."*
—Hodding Carter

Every child deserves to be treated as a worthy, valuable individual deserving of the utmost consideration and respect, but unfortunately this is not the world in which we live. By helping a child, whether your own or someone else's, you also help yourself through the resulting experience of immense satisfaction and joy that also serves to heighten your vibrational frequency. Children teach us valuable lessons as we observe their innocence, openness, freshness, lack of judgment, and curiosity, including the way they marvel at the smallest things.

Teaching Our Children to Live with Certainty

Your children will benefit immensely from learning early how to live with certainty. Research shows that older children and young adults with spiritual beliefs are happier, better performers, as well as more stable. Helping our children to become cognizant of what makes them happy, sad, mad, joyous, and passionate is a gift. Learning the basic tenets of Living with Certainty can even help them academically, as they'll learn to work hard at the things they love and to co-create their best life from a very young age.

Though specific circumstances, of course, come into play, most children are pure, open, untouched, and unaffected. They haven't yet been conditioned or jaded by the negativity of the ego-personality. For them, anything is possible. To thrive, our children need us to be positive role models, and to provide our love, presence, companionship, support, supervision, direction, and guidance.

The extent to which you believe in your own potential or limits is likely based on what you were told and what you observed as a child. Whether you have a victim mentality, or instead believe in your limitless potential, all started with your early conditioning. Don't pass any of your own limiting beliefs on to your children. Thinking, believing, and acting that your own potential is without limits sets the best possible example for your children. If your children consistently watch you swinging for the fences, they, too, will learn to think big and go for it in their own lives.

It's our responsibility to instill values, and then allow our children to make up their own minds and form their own opinions about things; to create a loving home environment that nourishes and provides safety, shelter, and security; to foster an open, exploring, and curious mind; to show them that this is an abundant universe without ceilings and limits; and to teach them gratitude. We must teach them that we're all interconnected, that everyone is uniquely different, and that this diversity is a wonderful aspect of life. Providing our children with boundaries also helps them to feel safe and secure. Through example, we can teach them how to live the life the universe always intended for them to live and experience deep-soul joy.

The family home should warmly welcome and embrace your children in a nest of joy, safety, sincerity, laughter, and possibility. Together the family unit should experience all life has to offer—sharing in both the best and the worst of times—while always treating each other with respect and affection. Family should provide us with a lifelong sense of connection, loyalty, unconditional love, acceptance, and belonging. Being raised in such fertile soil makes it easier to embrace our interconnectivity and extend ourselves with love and compassion as we grow older.

The Search Institute's Healthy Kids Initiative nicely sums up what is expected of parents: "Show Kids You Care: Notice them; Listen to them; Ask them about themselves; Encourage them to think big; Welcome their suggestions; Tell them how much you like being with them; Cheer their accomplishments; Keep promises you make; Answer their questions; Praise more, criticize less; Let them make mistakes; Make decisions together; Believe what they say; Encourage them to help others; Help them take a stand and stand with them; Let them tell you how they feel; Trust them; Include them in conversations; Find a common interest; Help them learn something new."[17]

Your children must know that you have an unwavering belief in their abilities and potential before life tries to knock the stuffing out of them. Help every child who is a part of your life to feel valuable, and to discover their purposeful authenticity and deep-soul joy. As Maria Shriver put it, "We are all worthy—not because we've accomplished something or because we're part of a famous family. You're worthy if you don't make the team, if you get D's and F's, if you don't get into the best college. That belief is the greatest gift any parent can give his or her child."[18]

38. Teachers and Wise Counsel

"The art of teaching is the art of assisting discovery."
—Kahlil Gibran

We all benefit from having wise mentors and teachers in our lives. They are the people who inspire and encourage us to dig deep to discover our truest potential. They live lives of grace and joy. Look for mentors and role models who have already mastered what you want to know, or achieved what you want to achieve. Your teachers may include family members, religious leaders, therapists, counselors, educators, co-workers, friends, coaches, instructors, social workers, and so on.

Teachers provide us with valuable guidance, and help us to truly see a situation for what it is, rather than just through the lens of our emotions. Powerful teachers have a strong sense of who they are, including a strong sense of humility. They're not concerned about the impression they make on you, nor do they try to persuade or influence you. They communicate by offering ideas and alternatives, but never force their own agenda. They are phenomenal listeners who are authentic and aware. Their lives are expressions of their purposeful authenticity.

When you're with a spiritual teacher, feelings of self-consciousness may indicate your ongoing lack of authenticity in certain areas. Anytime you act without authenticity by putting on an act or show so that your teacher will view you in a particular light, your feelings are going to indicate to you that these are areas for further examination. Your teacher will serve as a mirror for you in this way. Some of our most influential teachers, though we may not realize it at the time, are the ones who bring conflict and ensuing powerful lessons to our lives. Who provokes you and tests your mettle? Who pulls you through the fire? Who inspires you to be your best self? Who restores your faith, quells your skepticism, and jump-starts your curiosity? Above all, your teachers will have the ability to help you work through your issues in your quest to live in alignment with your purposeful authenticity.

You may require more help than can effectively be provided by friends and family. These people may not be comfortable providing you with the depth of feedback that you need, or be equipped with the skills to provide you with the kind of help or support you require. If this is the case, consider seeing a therapist or joining a support group that can provide you with the appropriate level of advice and guidance that you may need. (Note: Be wary of "life coaches" who aren't educated, certified, experienced, and successful, or who haven't achieved for themselves any of the things that you want.)

39. Personal Power

"Yet the full life is tied up with a sense in which one is aware of his own power as a person; that is, the belief that one can control or influence one's life to some extent, that one can modify or redirect the forces about one, that there is some energy at one's disposal to do so ... . Call it naïve optimism, if you will, but it is the central humanistic virtue."
—Paul Kurtz

As you live with certainty, you accept and embrace the power and responsibility you possess to co-create your life. You'll find this personal power to be an incredibly liberating and life-altering realization that may even make you feel immediately inclined to make sweeping changes in your life. As you become more self-reliant and independent and begin living with purposeful authenticity, you'll experience more self-respect, self-love, and confidence. Beliefs become clearer, choices become easier, and speaking your truth becomes essential.

One of the first areas people typically assess in their lives once they accept their personal power is the people who surround them. You may begin to see the people in your life in a new light. As you embrace your personal power and grow more protective of your vibrational frequency, you may feel that you no longer need or can tolerate anyone's negative energy. Now that you feel more self-reliant and empowered, the tenor of relationships may change as you begin to see people quite differently. While change may be necessary in your life as you realign with your inspired soul-view, you are doing the right thing for yourself and others, as long as your choices align positively with your internal instruction system.

40. Harm No One

"What is the greatest power? The greatest power is the Creator. But if you want to know the greatest strength, that is gentleness."
—Leon Shenandoah

The people who make you the angriest can serve as your most influential teachers. These heated exchanges carry great potential for learning and enlightenment, because being easily offended and over-sensitive are self-limiting soft spots. These moments test you. You must rise to the occasion and respond with self-respect and dignity, while respecting the others who are involved. This requires taking the time to listen and being empathetic. Always remember that you are in control of your responses, both external and internal.

Living with Certainty requires that you learn to avoid conflict and confrontation by taking a different approach—one that doesn't hurt others. This takes discipline and restraint, but a significant internal shift takes place when you stop seeing people as being merely human, and begin to see them first as souls.

Making fun of others seems to make some people feel better about their own deficiencies. By finding fault with others, gossiping, and being judgmental, you are being destructive to yourself and others, adding static to your energy vibrations. Remember that you have no idea where others are in their own spiritual journeys, or what it is they need to learn.

Michael Berg, the ordained Rabbi, Kabbalah scholar, and noted spiritual leader, said, "Most of us don't give much thought to the things we say. We assume that once we've said something, it's over and done with. Spiritually, this is not true. Words are energy and they live on."[19] Berg maintains that if you're in a foul mood and just aren't sure why, you should consider your energy level and karma. Have you done something to harm, hurt, or criticize someone, thereby lowering your own vibrational frequency level? When you don't apologize or act contritely, this negative energy sticks with you and remains dense and low-vibrating. Anytime you discuss the shortcomings of others, you rouse damaging, negative forces within yourself, so limit your focus to the good. Never say anything behind someone else's back that you wouldn't say in front of them.

There is no peace, gratitude, or joy in rage. If you engage in these behaviors—even when feeling provoked—you lower your energy and are not living with certainty. The equation is quite simple: When you hurt others, you hurt yourself and lower your vibrational frequency; when you love others, you love yourself and raise your vibrational frequency.

Responding to Your Anger

Rather than argue with someone, make an effort to be calm and even-toned. Explain your position, without getting caught up in proving you're right. People who lash out and engage in conflict, or who speak to you with disrespect probably don't respect themselves.

Release the expectation that they will behave differently, and remind yourself that nothing about this person's viewpoint or existence is needed to validate any aspect of your life. Then step back and lower your emotional level by objectively considering what it is that you're meant to learn from this challenging encounter. Keep in mind that at the soul-level we are all connected, and the other person is in need of compassion.

It's easy to get defensive when you feel that you are being unfairly attacked, but it's lazy to give into anger. Slow down and breathe. Instead of reacting, hold yourself in the moment and experience it. If you can excuse yourself to go sit with stillness, meditate, or practice your Sacred Sevens, by all means, do so. Allow feelings of interconnectivity and empathy to arouse your compassion. If you can, you'll be able to continue to communicate in a healthy manner.

You may also find it remarkably helpful to *force* yourself to think a kind thought about this person. You'll immediately notice that this simple act raises your vibrational level, calms you down, and makes you feel better, putting you in a more productive mindset to diffuse the situation.

When you are kind and loving, you naturally meet a more loving environment. When you are stressed and hostile, you meet a stressed and hostile environment. This is karma and applies to everything you put out there into the world. You'll get more of what you give.

41. Your Ancestors
"To forget one's ancestors is to be a brook without a source, a tree without a root."
—Chinese Proverb

How much time do you spend contemplating, honoring, thanking, and learning about your ancestors? These people are an important part of you and your history, and they should be acknowledged and honored.

Many people before me have worked and fought hard so that I might have this glorious, rich life. The awakening for me came many years ago when I learned that my great-grandmother was sold into a labor contract in Canada when she was twelve years old. This heart-wrenching knowledge lit a fire under me to make something of myself and serve as a positive light in the world. In her honor, and in honor of all of my departed ancestors, I will continue to use my life to shine as brightly as possible.

Living with Certainty requires you to know your personal history. Thanks to the Internet, there are many ways to investigate your ancestry. Have you visited the towns, cities, and countries in which your ancestors lived? Do you know how these individuals made a living? If you're named after a relative, have you made a special effort to know or learn about that person? Do you know your ancestors' stories—their military service, accomplishments, religious beliefs, languages, traditions, and so on? As you learn the answers to some of these questions, you may experience a special connection with your ancestors.

The energy of our loved ones remains with us even after they pass. You should feel compelled to pay tribute to those who came before you, and honor them with tremendous gratitude for all they did to affect your life and that of the generations who followed them. None of us would have the lives we do, if not for those who came before. To let their memories fade away into the past is an injustice. Do you and your family honor your ancestors, or preserve their memory through any kind of ritual?

One of the traditions of Japanese Buddhists is Obon, typically celebrated for several days during the summer. Obon is a time to pray for and pay tribute to the peace and tranquility of ancestors who have passed on. The belief is that the souls of these ancestors return to their homes for this important family observance and reunion. Many people take vacation during Obon in order to attend the ceremonies in their hometowns. Houses are cleaned and decorated, and foods are prepared and offered to the spirits of the ancestors at family alters that are decorated with flowers, lanterns, incense, and burning candles. The family visits the graves of their ancestors to call them back home, and even lights fires in front of their homes to guide their ancestors. At the end of the celebration, some families use their lanterns to guide the ancestors back to their graves. Others light candles that are placed inside of paper lanterns and floated down a river and out to the ocean. The day concludes with a festive family feast.

There are many things you can do as a family to honor and memorialize your ancestors. Begin by sharing and documenting stories and memories with your children about their grandparents and other relatives. Sharing stories and recollections allows you to celebrate these lives while sending an important message to your children that the passing of a loved one is an intrinsic aspect of the cycle of life, and not something to be feared or silenced. Through cherished rituals, we honor the memories of our ancestors and allow those who have passed to remain a vital presence within the family.

42. Boundaries

"I draw circles and sacred boundaries about me;
fewer and fewer climb with me up higher and higher mountains.
I am building a mountain chain out of ever-holier mountains."
—Friedrich Nietzche

When you really know and accept who you are, you set limits around what's acceptable and what's not, what's enough and what's not, and what's right and what's wrong. These boundaries are a way to protect your attitude and state of mind as you work to maintain a high vibrational frequency level. Conversely, you no longer violate the boundaries that others have set for themselves, and you expect the same consideration in return. Setting and communicating boundaries makes our relationships stronger, healthier, and more respectful as we come to understand and respect one another's limits and comfort levels.

Many executives describe with tremendous regret and hostility the sacrifices they made and the sacred boundaries (for example, missing priceless family time) they violated for their employers, who ultimately had no appreciation. As you live with certainty, you must set boundaries around what is sacred to you. What are you willing to sacrifice and where you are unwilling to compromise? The sacrifices you feel you must make should be affirmed by your internal instruction system as essential in order for you to live a life that is an expression of your purposeful authenticity.

43. Pets
*"Until one has loved an animal,
a part of one's soul remains unawakened."
—Anatole France*

Research is showing us that the lucky pet owners of the world require fewer doctor visits. Studies have shown that owning a pet also reduces stress and mental suffering, and that pets provide comfort, company, and unconditional love.[20] They generally make us feel good and heighten our energy. Many people open up and let down their guard with their pets more so than with their human family. Though they may not be able to say "I love you" to a family member, they can tell their pets a dozen times a day how much they love them. Similarly, many people feel as if they can give freely of themselves to a pet, but find that they are not comfortable being this open and exposed with another person. We can learn much about ourselves from our relationships with our pets. They can illuminate our soft spots.

If you're able to share your home with a pet, and are willing to take on the commitment and responsibility of caring for one, it's a wonderful way to open yourself, and to develop a deep appreciation of the animals that are an essential aspect of our life in this universe.

If you're not interested in having a pet, ask yourself *why*. Is it merely the commitment, or is there an aspect of you that has a general disregard and disrespect for animals, or even nature? If the latter is the case, this is an area of yourself that you should examine. People who have never loved a pet—and who say they *don't get it*—are, however, lucky in one way, because they have an immense growth opportunity. They haven't yet experienced this innate, powerful connection to non-human energy, essence, and love. Caring for a member of another species is a powerful, life-expanding experience.

> ### Kristi's Power Enabler
> *All healthy human beings require and crave kinship and community. From your life's primary relationships, you should gain love, fulfillment, support, connection, significance, contribution, affirmation of shared values, and personal growth. A truly healthy relationship is one in which you support each other in your quest to create lives that express your purposeful authenticity. With the right support, your spiritual quest can be enlivened and strengthened by those closest to you. Make a concerted effort to surround yourself with winners—kindhearted people living joyous, purposeful lives who know who they are and where they are going. As you engage in developing and maintaining these types of relationships, you will be connecting, sharing love, and further discovering your own essence. Put forth a conscious effort to make your relationships as open, positive, supportive, loving, healing, and encouraging as possible. Relative to the most intense relationships in your life—whether positive or negative—remember that they can provide you with some of life's most profound lessons as well as with invaluable insight into yourself, your spirituality, your authenticity, and your soft spots.*

CHAPTER 17

Beliefs

"Nothing splendid has ever been achieved except by those who dared believe that something inside them was superior to circumstance."
—Bruce Barton

YOUR BELIEFS CREATE the foundation of your life. They live in your core and guide your life by inspiring your actions, attitudes, choices, and thoughts. Your *articulated* beliefs are those beliefs and values that you readily acknowledge and espouse. Your *implicit* beliefs are the deeply rooted beliefs and values that you may not be completely conscious of, which to a large extent drive your actions and behaviors. You may not even be aware of how these beliefs came to be.

Your behavior is one of the best indicators of your beliefs. If you repeatedly act in a particular manner, you are operating with underlying convictions that are at the root of your actions. What you believe determines whether you create a life that expresses your purposeful authenticity and enables you to experience abundance and deep-soul joy. The most fulfilled, joyous individuals enter into each day believing that something amazing and miraculous will happen. Always believing the best about your potentiality without any limits feels good, and adds a luminescent quality to you and your life.

When we truly believe something, we feel clear and certain and experience intense emotions that in turn create powerful energy vibrations. These vibrations interact with the creative energy plane, which only deals in limitless possibilities. Belief is the language of Source energy.

Living with Certainty

Your focused thoughts, emotions, and beliefs are a powerful trio. When they're all in alignment with your inspired soul-view, they produce powerful energy vibrations. The key is to gain control over them and leverage this power every day of your life. Through your own efforts to live with certainty you stimulate and galvanize idle energy to co-create a purposeful, joyous life. Complete and utter belief in your ability to co-create the life the universe always intended for you to live is your greatest single power.

As you live with certainty you must have a deep and unwavering belief and trust that you can and will leave behind the dysfunction of your ego-personality to discover your inspired soul-view; that Source energy is with you and guiding you at all times if you would just slow down and take notice; that you can and will create a life that is the fullest expression of your purposeful authenticity; that you can and will be provided with ample opportunities to experience the fulfillment and joy of serving others and making a unique contribution to the planet; and that you can and will experience deep-soul joy.

We Live in a Friendly Universe

You must believe and know that this is a loving, friendly, abundant, responsive, and gracious universe. Source energy exists only for good; there is no opposing evil or negative Source. With this belief comes an increase in signs, signals, symbols, and synchronicities that not only provide invaluable guidance, but also reinforce your belief about how the universe works and how you are loved. When you believe, as Einstein describes, that we live in a friendly universe, then you can trust that there is nothing inherently bad in the circumstances of your life; everything exists as it does to help you learn. With the belief that the universe is on your side, you can stop swimming against the current.

Our Core Beliefs Shape Us

We all hold certain core beliefs that shape who we are and form the basis for how we approach our choices and decisions. When your life circumstances are consistently difficult and challenging, it's time to examine any beliefs that may be creating static and holding you back. You may be attracting the wrong things through your thoughts, which are rooted at their foundation in your beliefs. Your core beliefs may be in conflict with your conscious beliefs.

These central beliefs are deeply embedded within your subconscious, and profoundly affect the creation of your reality. If you find that your life seems to be filled with the exact opposite of what you want, it may be because your core beliefs are influencing you in ways of which you're not even aware. Determine what your fundamental beliefs are by contemplating your passion and talents, greatest successes, soft spots, relationships, ability to love and be loved, spirituality and faith, commitment to truth, imagination and inspiration, values, early negative conditioning, tendencies to compare yourself to and judge others, feelings of envy and jealousy, ability to live with awareness, commitment to living authentically, and your level of courage.

To truly empower yourself, you must have a complete faith that the universe is a safe and loving place where joy and the expression of your truest self are the overarching purpose of life. You're only limited by your ability not to think big enough.

44. Conscious and Subconscious Beliefs

*"The mind is the limit. As long as the mind can envision the fact that you can do something, you can do it—
as long as you really believe 100%."*
—Arnold Schwarzenegger

The conscious part of your mind is alert and mentally aware of yourself as a thinking being. It knows what you're feeling and doing, and why. However, it can only process a fraction of what's happening around you. The subconscious part of your mind, on the other hand, lies just below the level of awareness of the conscious mind, and is not immediately available to your consciousness.

Your subconscious is attuned to and registers—as if keeping a log—every aspect of your life and surroundings, including the emotions and energy of the people around you. The experiences and feelings of your entire lifetime are stored in your subconscious. They have the power to sabotage your efforts to live with certainty if the dysfunctional parts are not identified and eliminated, as they play a significant role in shaping how you see yourself. You likely have some self-limiting behaviors and beliefs deeply rooted in your subconscious. These may include addiction, co-dependency, a tendency to be overcritical, or feelings of victimization.

You may not even be aware of negative or self-limiting subconscious beliefs. If, however, you routinely catch yourself engaging in unhealthy thoughts or behaviors, you may need to transform your subconscious mind to a more positive, healthy state. If negative thoughts catch your attention, stop and acknowledge what you're doing and feeling. Allow yourself to experience the emotion. What is your internal instruction system telling you to do? How does your energy feel? Are you vibrating at a high frequency? Are you proud of your thoughts and actions—or would you be embarrassed if others knew? Is this behavior representative of who you are and who you want to be?

Affirmations, meditation, gratitude, and visualizations can help weaken limiting, self-conscious beliefs by using your conscious mind to reprogram your subconscious mind. When you feel safe, secure, loved, and trusted—and extend that love and trust to others—your subconscious mind feels the freedom to ease up.

45. Faith and Trust

"My faith is brightest in the midst of impenetrable darkness."
—Mohandas K. Gandhi

Faith is having complete conviction, belief, and trust in the truth, value, or trustworthiness of a person, idea, or thing without needing logical proof or material evidence. It's an optimistic, hopeful approach to life that allows you to trust in Source energy because even though you can't see it, you can feel it. Faith is awareness of the Source energy within, and encompasses your intuition, inspiration, and vision. Abraham Joshua Heschel said, "Faith is the beginning of compassion, of compassion for God."[21] With faith you can let go of the need to control and orchestrate every aspect of your life. With faith, you will experience more of the peace you deserve. The test of faith is to trust that there is more to our existence than this Earthly physicality; that something bigger, a universal intelligence, transcends all that we think we know.

Faith is unshakeable; you either have it or you don't. It allows you to operate from the place of knowing that irrespective of what happens, you will be fine, and that you aren't walking through this journey alone. Source energy is within you, working with you at all times to co-create your life. With faith, you'll no longer question the veracity of your internal instruction system or other guidance received through signs, signals, symbols, or synchronicities. When you understand that this guidance will always be there for you, you'll feel significant relief—as if you can finally exhale.

46. Limitless Abundance and Your Dreams

"The dreamer and his dreams are the same ...
the powers personified in a dream are those that move the world."
—Joseph Campbell

As you align with your purposeful authenticity, think big and ask for everything you want in prayer. Visualize, fantasize, and dream about your soul-view–aligned desires. Embrace new approaches that may be pathways to the next level. In life, as you enter one door, there's always a next level to achieve.

Possibilities abound—Living with Certainty will teach you to leverage your power to explore these possibilities. To live with certainty, you must think, feel, believe, and act from a mindset of abundance, even before this becomes an Earthly reality. Becoming abundant internally helps to fuel change, raise your vibrational frequency, and create external abundance in your life.

Keep in mind that abundance in your life does not necessarily translate directly to money, because money may not be what's needed for you to experience deep-soul joy. Abundance can appear in your life in a number of other ways, including opportunities. Until you discover and align with your inspired soul-view, you may continue to believe that you won't really live or be happy until the money shows up. This is only societal conditioning, and your ego exerting its influence.

Would you rather live a life of deep-soul joy or would you rather have money and be miserable? This isn't to say you can't have both—of course you can. But money can no longer be your only goal. Money alone does not create deep-soul joy; only the purposeful activity that led to the creation of the money can create deep-soul joy. When you experience internal abundance and joy, external abundance follows.

47. Receptivity

"Make your ego porous. Will is of little importance, complaining is nothing, fame is nothing. Openness, patience, receptivity, solitude is everything."
—Rainer Maria Rilke

You must feel open, receptive, and worthy of receiving the experience of deep-soul joy and the life the universe always intended for you to live. You must feel deserving of all of the blessings, goodness, grace, and lessons that come your way. We have already discussed how gratitude helps to facilitate this, but receptivity and anticipation are also powerful feelings. Being open and anticipating that goodness will fill your life allows you to vibrate energy at a high frequency. As your desires manifest themselves, give thanks and move on to anticipating and being receptive of the next great thing.

In the past, when I experienced a synchronistic event I used to make the mistake of saying, "Wow, isn't that wild? Can you believe that happened?" I know now that this response sent a message to the universe that I was in disbelief—that I felt that this was an unusual, extraordinary event. I now anticipate that the universe will operate precisely as I've outlined in these pages, and I simply give great thanks for these mini-miracles.

48. Visualization

"In visualization, we expand what we have by expanding what we want."
—Adelaide Bry

Visualization enables you to see yourself as already living the life of your dreams and having the things you want. You focus your thoughts on detailed, vivid pictures that provoke an emotional and physical response that create feelings of having already achieved your desires, already living the life of your dreams. Think of it as watching a personal movie about your life. Visualization helps you along in your effort to co-create the life the universe always intended for you to live by inspiring and motivating you.

If this seems foreign to you, think again. Have you never daydreamed? Fundamentally, the mind constructs and responds to visual images. Human societies have constructed words and language as a means of communicating with one another. Our minds, however, communicate powerfully with us through visual images. Many world-class athletes routinely utilize the visualization of every aspect of their event, course, or race as part of their training. If visualization is a worthwhile technique for Olympians to help them achieve their goals, it's worth trying yourself.

Your subconscious mind cannot differentiate between whether you're actually experiencing an event, or just imagining it. The subconscious reacts to mental stimuli and experiences visualizations as if they are true, real events. This is good news, because by visualizing your goals, you program your subconscious mind to begin performing to its fullest potential and working toward making your visions manifest in your life.

It can be very powerful and helpful to create a vision book or vision board that reflects precisely the vision you see in your mind. Create a collage comprised of pictures and photos—from magazines, books, newspapers, and other sources—that represent your soul-view–aligned desires. These images should stimulate and inspire you, and represent the life the universe always intended for you to live. Include inspirational quotes and personal affirmations. The content will change over time as you achieve various goals. Spend time at the beginning and end of each day with your vision book/board. Seeing your dreams in this level of detail—even writing out every detail in a journal—allows you to experience the feelings of the soul-view–aligned life that you are working so hard to co-create.

While visualization does not require hypnosis, it has the most impact when you find a quiet location where you can get comfortable, close your eyes, and focus your breath. As you clear your mind and achieve a relaxed state, begin imagining yourself living the soul-view–aligned life of your dreams. Picture colors, sounds, smells, and conversations. How does the day start? Where are you? What do you see? What do you hear? What are you doing? Who are you with and how are you interacting with them? What are you eating? What are you wearing? What are you feeling (this is the most significant aspect of the visualization)?

Repeat to yourself that you deserve this desire, that it's an aspect of your inspired soul-view, and that it's on its way to being made manifest in your life. The more realistic and detailed the images, the more credence and impact it will have on your subconscious mind. Go deep and internalize the feelings of already having achieved your goals. Do this several times a day to align your mind and your body in co-creation.

49. Hope

"Hope is the dream of a soul awake."
—French Proverb

Hope allows you to desire something with the confident expectation of its fulfillment. Hope gives you promise for the future. Intense hope is knowledge accompanied by euphoria-like feelings of the future manifestation of your potential. A joyful life has a strong foundation rooted in hope.

Hope, however, isn't a plan; we must separately commit to growth and development. Henry David Thoreau stated, "If you have built castles in the air, your work need not be lost; that is where they should be. Now put the foundations under them." Your intentions and inspired soul-view–aligned actions must be used to prepare and propel you into the right circumstances and direction. What are you hoping for? What are you willing to work for?

50. Convictions

"Strong convictions precede great actions. The man strongly possessed by an idea is the master of all who are uncertain or wavering. Clear, deeply held convictions rule the world."
—James Freeman Clark

Your convictions are your most unshakable beliefs. When your soul-view alignment and the desire to express your purposeful authenticity are backed up by a strong will and the mental determination to achieve your desires, you are a powerhouse. A passionate and strong will keeps your focus on the prize. Your possibilities and potential are endless because abundance knows no bounds.

Most people who have "made it" are no more gifted or endowed than those who just can't seem to catch a break. However, they possess the dream, belief, conviction, iron will, drive, and determination that others lack. Once you discover your purposeful authenticity and set a vision for yourself to the point that you can see and feel it, your will and discipline keep your mind set on actualizing the vision. Possessing the will to create the life the universe always intended for you to live is a big part of the battle. While this is simple in theory, the required clarity and discipline can be difficult to achieve.

A word of caution about conviction: Having an iron will isn't a good thing when it's actually your ego trying to seize control from the peaceful faith of your inspired soul-view. This is a misuse of power. As you live with certainty, you may need to bend and surrender, as we have discussed, to remain open and in the flow of your spiritual power frequency. Remember, the goal is to keep your energy vibrating at a high level. When you feel the need to force and control, you'll no longer feel good, and it's a sign that you're vibrating dense, low-frequency energy. However, when a strong will helps to keep you committed to manifesting your inspired soul-view–aligned goals, it is a good and necessary thing.

51. Expectations

"High achievement always takes place in the framework of high expectation."
—Charles F. Kettering

While we must learn to expect soul-view–aligned goodness to grace our lives, we must not become so attached to non-soul-view–aligned expectations that we allow ourselves to become devastated if our expectations are dashed. Be very careful not to cling too closely to certain outcomes, particularly those that are not aligned with your inspired soul-view—because when they don't materialize, you may feel that you have somehow failed.

A lot of anger, frustration, and resentment result from not getting what you want. These are dangerous feelings, because they ultimately serve to keep what you want at bay. By creating static through the pain of dashed expectations, you impede the universe from delivering what it is that you really *need*.

Many of us make the mistake of becoming attached to non-soul-view–aligned expectations and outcomes that never come to fruition. Then we get stuck, lowering our vibrational frequency and making ourselves feel bad. Remember to remain open, flowing, and receptive to what comes. As co-creator of your life, you must surrender old notions about expectations to your inspired soul-view. It's only your ego that causes you to hang tightly to specific unrealistic expectations and outcomes.

Remember, too, that you cannot dream too big or hope too much. Expect Living with Certainty to expand your life to the fullest representation of the life the universe always intended for you to live. Expect that you will discover and align with your inspired soul-view. Expect that you will create a life that is the fullest expression of your purposeful authenticity. Expect that through your unique attributes and gifts, you will be of immense service to the world. Expect the magic, guidance, and grace of the universe to touch your life every day through signs, signals, symbols, and synchronicities. Expect that your internal instruction system will provide you with guidance that will never lead you astray. Expect deep-soul joy.

> ## Kristi's Power Enabler
> *Where are you limiting yourself? Is it possible that your beliefs are not at all aligned with your inspired soul-view? Your personal identity is wrapped up in your beliefs which can at times be negative and destructive forces in your life as they vibrate powerful energy out to the universe. You cannot align with the flow of your spiritual power frequency or positively co-create your life when your foundational beliefs are that of uncertainty, hopelessness, limits, cynicism, and doubt. Never focus on the prospect of failure. And never tell yourself that your dreams are too lofty. You will ultimately make manifest a life that is in accordance with your core beliefs, so if you want to co-create and attract different circumstances, you have to change your core beliefs. This may require letting go of needless boundaries and limits you have set for yourself or had conditioned into your psyche at any early age.*
>
> *Once you realize that you are, in fact, the one who has limited your own life and circumstances through the beliefs you hold about yourself, you can begin to unshackle yourself from these limits. As you embrace the fact that a life of purposeful authenticity and deep-soul joy is well within your grasp, you will begin to take control of your life in a way that you never have before.*

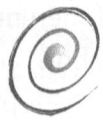

CHAPTER 18

Gratitude

*"Imagine an ox's yoke adrift / On the vast ocean and a turtle
Happening to poke its head / Through the hole—
This is how rare / And extraordinary it is to
Be born a human being."*
—Kunkhyen Longchen Rabjam

GRATITUDE DOESN'T REQUIRE a particular faith or religious practice, but just simple feelings of genuine thankfulness for who you are, what you have, and where you are in your life. Gratitude is an act of integrity without negativity, judgment, or static. It is a loving mindset and perspective. It has been well documented that an attitude of gratitude lends itself to better overall mental and physical health. Living with a heart full of gratitude, generosity, and joy creates a full life—one of constant blessings and grace.

Gratitude changes your energy. As you express heartfelt gratitude and appreciation to the universe, you create an optimal vibration that aligns with Source energy and, in turn, attracts more blessings, grace, and abundance into your life. Your goal must be to double-triple-quadruple the amount of time you have spent in your life up until now in a state of heartfelt gratitude. It is astounding how the consistent vibration of energy at this high frequency level can transform your life. When times are tough, or you catch yourself thinking a negative thought, transcend the moment by giving heartfelt thanks for some other aspect of your life. This simple act changes your mindset while purifying and heightening your energy.

The energy of gratitude and love are as close as humans can get to Source energy. Gratitude is a direct exchange of love and thankfulness between you and the universe, and is an essential aspect of Living with Certainty. By being thankful to the universe for what you have and what you are about to receive, you acknowledge your unwavering faith that something out there is working out of pure love on your behalf.

Use your first waking moments each day to be thankful for your breath and your life. Use this time to vibrate the high frequency energies that you intend to fill your day. Don't squander this brief and essential time by jumping into thinking, planning, and worrying about mundane activities. There will always be time for that. Instead, meet the new day with a fresh, blank slate of gratitude-laden, high-vibrational energy emanating from the sweet clarity with which you awaken.

Up until now you may have taken your life's difficult circumstances into consideration and felt that you have little for which to be grateful. However, if you are truly to transition your mind and your life through Living with Certainty, you must spend as much of your time as possible in the high-vibrational state of gratitude. Quite simply, not appreciating your life is devaluing it. Remain cognizant every day of the big and little things that make you smile, lighten your load, teach you a lesson, or bring a fleeting feeling of joy. The only way to make gratitude a fundamental aspect of your being is to heighten your awareness and develop the habit of expressing thanks for your life in its entirety, just as it exists today.

No matter how bad you may think your circumstances are, someone always has it worse than you, and life can be taken from you in the blink of an eye. Anything this fragile and fleeting must be cared for, revered, and appreciated. The more you accept and internalize this fact, the more gratitude you will express for who you are and what you have today.

There are many things to be grateful for—the smiles and greetings of strangers; books and music; the warm afternoon sun; the renewal and safety of last night's sleep; the warmth of your fireplace; the magnificence of a ripe, summer peach; the shade of a tree on a hot day; pure drinking water; your child's safety; the love of friends; the walk you took through the park; the hummingbird that fluttered by your hanging pot; the learning that came from a difficult circumstance; freedom; and so on. As simple as some of these things are, never take them for granted. Millions of people around the world do not have the most basic of these things.

52. Appreciation

*"It isn't the great pleasures that count the most;
it's making a great deal out of the little ones."*
—Jean Webster

Here's a radical idea: On a regular basis, be appreciative for every aspect of your life—every person, circumstance, soft spot, and lesson. By appreciating someone—even a *difficult* someone—we show that we are aware of them and value them. We demonstrate that we respect them enough to be sensitive to them, show them our gratitude, and hold them dear. The simple act of appreciation has the power to completely change your perspective on your current circumstances, as well as the effect they have on developing and shaping you.

Overtly showing your appreciation to loved ones, friends, co-workers, acquaintances, and even strangers is a very potent way to strengthen relationships and to extend more positive, loving energy out into the universe. Everyone needs to feel appreciated. Everyone. *Isn't it ironic that we very often treat those closest to us with the least respect and regard?* We somehow find the energy to put on a kind face for strangers, but not those closest to us.

Reveal your appreciative, kinder side to everyone—but most *certainly* to your family and inner circle. Express your appreciation in a million different ways for their presence and support in your life. As you open your heart this way, you become better, kinder, more loving, generous, and grateful. As you live with more love and gratitude, you also purify and heighten your energy vibrations and intensify your own deep-soul joy. You have a lifelong obligation to care for those closest to you. How do you show them how much they mean to you? What are you doing to show your inner circle how much you love them?

53. Count Your Blessings Every Day

"We can only be said to be alive in those moments when our hearts are conscious of our treasures."
—Thornton Wilder

Give thanks every day for all that you have. Try this upon waking in the morning and going to bed at night. Actually say, *Thank you for all of the blessings in my life*. Begin and end each day in a peaceful, righteous place of gratitude. Be aware of what you have that makes you happy and what you have that you love. Thank the universe daily for these things.

Your attitude and perspective are important. Every day, you have the option to thank the universe for what you do have—versus placing focus on that which you don't have. Your life is 25 percent about what happens to you and 75 percent about your reaction. Make a choice to focus your energy on all that is right with your life through immense, daily gratitude, and you'll find that more of your soul's deepest desires will eventually be made manifest through your passionate, purpose-fueled actions.

54. Grace and Reverence

"There is a built-in sense of indebtedness in the consciousness of man, an awareness of owing gratitude, of being called upon at certain moments to reciprocate, to answer, to live in a way which is compatible with the grandeur and mystery of living."
—Abraham Joshua Heschel

You receive kindness and compassion every day from Source energy. Think of those times when you've made a mistake or a bad decision, and yet the sky didn't fall in on you. When you get a pass like this from the universe, allow it to humble you—and then give great thanks. This grace should inspire you to be more understanding, forgiving, and compassionate toward others who are just as humanly frail and prone to mistakes as you are. This is called grace.

As you live with certainty, you live from a place of honor and respect for the universe, and will experience a gentler, more loving universe than you previously perceived. With reverence, you see beyond the surface of the physical world and have a clear sense of the underlying energy, mystery, and love that is present for all of us. You understand that life is a sacred gift, and come to respect and appreciate this time you have in Earthly physicality.

Every aspect of the universe is a miraculous gift. Stare out at the infinite blackness at night with curiosity and reverence. Feel how small and interconnected we all are. This type of deep, spiritual contemplation will give you a new appreciation for a bird's nest or a mighty oak tree. If you really have reverence for life in all of its forms, you'll never again see another living thing as less than you. Everything has intrinsic value. With reverence, you are compassionate, connected, and kind. You cannot harm, damage, or devastate. Begin living with a greater respect and reverence for every aspect of our universe. Smell a flower, take in the blue sky, rejoice in the rain, catch a snowflake, watch a bird eating a worm, and stop deliberately stepping on bugs when you take your daily walk. Every little thing you do and tell yourself counts. Live with reverence for all.

55. Celebrations

*"The more you praise and celebrate your life,
the more there is in life to celebrate."*
—Oprah Winfrey

Celebrating and honoring yourself is not an egotistical act; it's a loving one. Acknowledge and mark your accomplishments all throughout your life. Sometimes these may be private celebrations to reward yourself for your progress, commitment, discipline, or breakthroughs. At other times, you may invite others to share in your joy. Do the same for others—as you witness those closest to you passing milestones or doing great things, honor them and celebrate with them.

Make celebration in tandem with gratitude a consistent ritual in your life. Balloons, cake, and party favors? Only if that's what you want. Maybe treating yourself to a massage or a luxurious, candlelit bubble bath sounds better, or perhaps enjoying an exceptional glass of wine sipped under the stars, or buying yourself an exotic plant, is exactly the reward you desire. Whatever you choose, make sure it has meaning, and helps to heighten the energy within you and your environment. Honor, celebrate, and rejoice in your life, its blessings, and your forward movement. Savor the moments that mark your progress. Deliberately create celebratory moments and memories as you co-create the life the universe always intended for you to live. Keep the spirit of celebration and gratitude alive in all of your life.

56. Giving and Generosity
"They who give have all things; they who withhold have nothing."
—Hindu Proverb

Not only is it essential that you give thanks, but you must also return kindness and live with generosity. Gratitude and generosity are nearly one and the same, and both play powerful roles in heightening your energy vibrations and intensifying your spiritual power frequency. Any time you receive, make it a point to give. Pass on a gift wherever and whenever you can. Think of yourself as a bottomless well, an Earthly source of all that is good, right, and abundant. From this place, give to the world with the noble intention of spreading joy and making the world a better place.

Giving and love are two of the primary sources of life's greatest joys. Giving for no reason other than you want to share of yourself feels the best. Giving takes on special meaning and authenticity when you share the things that you love with the people you care about and love the most. Give treasures and gifts with a story—items that will trigger people to think of you and the treasured times you have spent together. Unique gifts given from the heart that remind someone of a special moment in time mean the most. The gifts you give should be as authentic as the individuals to whom you are giving, and can include anything that is special to you or that you know will create a meaningful experience for the recipient. Giving *always* feels great.

57. Rituals

*"Every morning, our first thought should be
a wish to devote the day to the good of all living beings."*
—Dilgo Khyentse Rinpoche

Rituals are part of an established routine done at regular intervals, and can include anything that you feel assists in summoning that which is sacred to you. Rituals help us to mark sacred events and benchmarks, and help to perpetuate connectivity and community. Incorporate rituals and practices into your life to help foster your spiritual awakening and summon your inspired soul-view.

Rituals are most powerfully observed as a daily practice. Designate a peaceful, sacred space for yourself where you are surrounded with things that will create strong, positive spiritual energy for you. Tools that encourage connection to Spirit include gongs, statues, mantras, candles, incense, music, poetry, crucifixes, the rosary, mandalas, prayer beads, and inspirational quotes, or activities such as dancing, deep breathing, yoga, chanting, fasting, and praying. Each of these has an amazing capacity to align us with our inspired soul-view. Each of these may affect you differently, so experiment to see which are the most inspirational for you personally. Music, for instance, may have a calming effect on one person and yet be disruptive for another. Through trial and error, figure out what works best for you.

58. Honor and Commemorate

*"If you're respectful by habit, constantly honoring the worthy,
four things increase: long life, beauty, happiness, and strength."*
—Buddha

Tokens, mementos, keepsakes, and remembrances all serve to remind you of the significant and powerful times you have spent alone or with a loved one. They serve as visual reminders of happy events or moments for which you should be eternally grateful.

Take the time and put forth the energy to honor, commemorate, and memorialize people and life events that you never want to forget. You can do this in a variety of ways, including assembling photo albums and scrapbooks, or documenting events in a journal devoted to special memories. Store photos, rocks, charms, or crystals gathered during meaningful moments in a lovely memento box. Do what you can to maintain the positive energy of these memories in a way that brings back vivid details of these special moments.

Anytime you feel restless, anxious, or sleepless, summon cherished memories of your happiest times and allow them to float through your mind. Maybe these are family camping trips you took as a child, special vacations, times spent with family members and pets, gardens you created, holidays, or sporting events. Time spent focusing on happy memories puts us in a very peaceful and fulfilled place in our minds. Give thanks for all of these cherished memories that continue to bring you joy.

Kristi's Power Enabler

An entitlement mindset has overtaken much of America, particularly the younger generations. Feeling entitled is ego-driven and one of the worst ways to move through life. Allowing your heightened awareness to help you develop a natural inclination to recognize and show appreciation for all acts of grace, guidance, and kindness is the only answer. As it pertains to Living with Certainty, I am prescribing a ceaseless mindset of thanks—an overwhelming "can't-contain-yourself, yell-from-the rooftop" feeling of gratefulness as opposed to mere fleeting moments of gratitude that inspire you to write a thank-you note or jot a note in your journal (which is a great way to develop a gratitude habit, but cannot be the end goal). Gratitude is a foundational approach to life for some of the most joyful, tranquil, compassionate, and generous people I know—it is how they connect to the universe on a moment-to-moment basis. Heartfelt gratitude immediately transforms your energy to high-frequency vibrations that are in alignment with Source energy. Think of gratitude as the ultimate means of tapping into you spiritual power frequency so that you may receive more of the life the universe always intended for you to live.

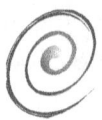

CHAPTER 19

Progress

*"'How does one become a butterfly?' she asked pensively.
'You must want to fly so much that you are willing
to give up being a caterpillar.'"*
—Trina Paulus

BY NOW, YOU UNDERSTAND that you have sole Earthly responsibility for your life. All this book can provide for you is a guide, or template, to change your life. The journey to personal spiritual enlightenment requires your valiant, ongoing courage and commitment as you allow yourself to become aware, honest, unguarded, exposed, sincere, and receptive.

Without discipline and accountability, you'll settle back into familiar patterns. When you're not feeling joyous, enlivened, hopeful, or inspired, and are not experiencing flow or any signs, signals, symbols, and synchronicities, it's a clear indication that you're not vibrating at a pure, high frequency level and are not aligned with the flow of your spiritual power frequency. With some introspection, you may very well find that you have not been living fully in accordance with the Living with Certainty tenets and Energy Enablers. This is the time to regroup, reread this book, rededicate to your meditation practice, and assess where you have gotten off-track.

If you desire real and lasting change, you'll have to significantly change how you've been living. Let's be realistic—it may take the remainder of your lifetime to undo the unhealthy conditioning which has prevented you from discovering and knowing your essence. Living with certainty is not a goal with set timetables and deadlines, but a lifelong process.

Over time, however, little changes result in big transformation.

You must stick with this program for at least six weeks, which is the minimum amount of time it will take to begin establishing new patterns, control your self-talk, and try new behaviors that may run counter to a lifetime of conditioning. You may need to give up the "you" who you thought you were, and begin the difficult task of climbing out of your comfort zone. If you are to develop new patterns, you must work through this tension with perseverance. Each time that you persevere through this type of discomfort, you grow.

You will successfully live with certainty when the Energy Enablers come naturally and no longer feel merely like a prescription from a book. Over time, living with certainty will become an authentic, easy, and natural way to approach your life and spirituality. You'll grasp the profundity of the term "spirituality-as-lifestyle" as your soul-view more frequently and easily becomes available and accessible to you. As the inner volume of your soul turns up, the outer static will fade into the background.

Every morning, begin your day by encouraging yourself to remain awake, aware, inquisitive, and open to life's experiences. As you close your day, mentally walk through its events and your reactions. Where did you stick to your principles or follow your instinct? Where did you experience bad feelings? Where did you resist or deny? Where did you hurt or help? Where did you create static or close down? These questions help to hold you accountable, and the answers will provide the fodder for additional work and introspection.

59. Legacy

"I may be here for a short while, gone tomorrow into oblivion or until the days come to take me away. But, in whatever part you play, be remembered as part of a legacy ... of sharing dreams and changing humanity for the better. It's that legacy that never dies."
—Author unknown

What are you going to hand down to future generations? What indelible mark are you making on the world? We are remembered for our inspired, original actions and achievements. What do you want to be remembered for as a human being? Serving others and sharing your gifts create a legacy and an example for all to follow.

Your legacy may be as simple as having offspring whom you love and adore, and who love and adore you in return. Whatever your legacy will be, it will be built one inspired soul-view–aligned day, action, and choice at a time. You may worry that you won't find your purpose or relevancy before you die. Living with Certainty should eliminate that worry, because you're now well on your way. What will your contribution be?

60. Endurance

"Endurance is not just the ability to bear a hard thing, but to turn it into glory."
—William Barclay

Endurance gives you the power to withstand hardship because you want something badly. There is no greater aspiration than to discover your inspired soul-view, to create a life that is the fullest expression of your purposeful authenticity, and to live every day with deep-soul joy. As strongly as you may desire these things in your life, however, go easy on yourself—you're an apprentice in the Living with Certainty practice.

Even when you really want to change your life, it takes tremendous commitment and drive to keep on going. No change happens overnight. Your feelings about the quality of your life and your circumstances aren't going to change in any meaningful way until you begin the internal work needed to believe, feel, and act differently. This is hard work that requires commitment and stamina. It is well worth the effort, though, because you'll discover in short order that you're able to cope with the ups and downs of life more effectively and gracefully. Once you begin to live a life that is an expression of your purposeful authenticity and begin moving forward through soul-view–aligned action, you'll be so infused with purpose that you'll have the motivation to keep going. Let nothing keep you from the life the universe always intended for you to live.

61. Evolution, Transformation, and Becoming

*"Personal transformation can and does have global effects.
As we go, so goes the world, for the world is us.
The revolution that will save the world is ultimately a personal one."*
—Marianne Williamson

We are wired to know when it's time for transformation—we experience longing, dullness, agitation, and impatience. Very often, however, it takes more than just those feelings to push us forward. We may need a crisis or calamity to shake us awake and alert us to the fact that we must change.

Living with Certainty will cause you to view yourself and your life differently. It's as if up until now, you have been living with your face planted in the wide end of a funnel, looking at a view that's severely narrow and limited in scope. Living with Certainty immediately rights things by turning that funnel around so that you can begin enjoying a far more expansive view. Love, service, and peace will become the foundational states from which you live and never want to leave. This is a time of transformation for you. Through Living with Certainty, your possibility and potential are now probability. You've been given the information and tools; it's now up to you to commit, to act, and to believe in yourself.

62. Patience

*"Be patient toward all that is unsolved in your heart and try to love
the questions themselves. Do not now seek the answers,
which cannot be given you because you would not be able to live them.
And the point is to live everything. Live the questions."*
—Rainier Maria Rilke

The events of the life the universe always intended for you to live unfold when and how they should, when you are ready. Only Source energy knows your full potential, and how things should unfold in order for you to learn the lessons that will prepare you for the unfurling of your true potential. Nothing is revealed until you can handle it.

As a co-creator, but not the sole creator of your life, you can't control the pace of change, manifestation, and forward movement. Living with Certainty requires that you have faith that you're on track, and that you muster the patience to accept that things are unfolding in the exact way and time that's required.

Patience and good-natured tolerance are useful traits to develop in yourself. Impulsive, rash action always results in the most reckless results and consequences. You will undoubtedly react more thoughtfully and in an inspired soul-view–aligned manner when you slow down and practice patience.

63. Prioritization
"Getting in touch with your true self must be your first priority."
—Tom Hopkins

How you spend your time and what you focus on is a choice you make daily. You must be extremely protective of your time. It is imperative that you prioritize and focus your time and effort on what will yield the greatest dividends. What are the most significant and critical activities that you must undertake in order to reach your goals? Where do you need to develop relationships? What skills do you need to acquire? These are the things that should fill your calendar. As you take action to co-create a life that is the fullest possible expression of your purposeful authenticity, frequently ask yourself what needs to be completed each day to keep the ball moving forward.

64. Humor
*"Humor is an affirmation of dignity,
a declaration of man's superiority to all that befalls him."*
—Romain Gary

Humor, when it is not at someone else's expense, is an effective means of being kinder and gentler to yourself. It feels good and raises your personal vibrational frequency. It provides you with the ability to lighten up and stop taking yourself so seriously. Humor also helps to take the sting out of difficult moments, and helps to transition your energy to a higher vibrational frequency. What would happen if you didn't take yourself so seriously and stopped making mountains out of molehills? Can you lighten up and just go with the flow? The answer is *yes, you can,* and it may be high time that you gave yourself a break.

You don't have to be happy-go-lucky every moment of the day, but you don't need to be intensely serious, either. No matter what is happening around you, you'll enjoy yourself, others, and your environment more if you maintain a sense of humor. The higher your confidence and self-esteem, the easier it is to laugh at yourself. Be spontaneous—you have to break out of predictable reactions to lighten up. Make the choice to let go of things that really aren't important, and stop thinking that your entire sense of self is somehow wrapped up in objectives that are in no way aligned with your inspired soul-view. Very often, the mundane events of your life are worthy of humor— many of them are ultimately transactions and not nearly as dramatic as you might think.

65. Freedom

"Everything can be taken from a man but one thing: the last of the human freedoms—to choose one's attitude in any given set of circumstances, to choose one's own way."
—Victor Frankl

As Deepak Chopra so wisely observed, "Every human being is in search of freedom—freedom from worry, freedom from illness, freedom from confusion, freedom from a sense of isolation."[22] Freedom feels good to us. This is why we universally seek it. What we don't generally understand is that this type of freedom is a choice. As we choose to live a purposeful life, we are free—and there's no more natural way to heighten your energy and experience the joy of freedom than to live a life that expresses your purposeful authenticity.

Your biggest freedom is that which allows you to make the choices that determine how you feel and how you will shape your life. You are free to discover and co-create the life the universe always intended for you to live in alignment with your inspired soul-view. This freedom allows for creativity, inspiration, and joy—though you remain accountable for your choices and decisions.

You may, at times, find freedom disconcerting. The pressure and anxieties you previously experienced over pleasing others, competing, and living an inauthentic life can become deeply conditioned into your beings. Once this weight is lifted, you feel very different as you become free to act and react in accordance with your internal instruction system.

You cannot rise up to your truest self without honesty, truth, and self-love. Living with truth means that you no longer pretend to be someone you are not, nor do you dwell on what other people think. With truth comes authentic personal power and freedom. No longer consumed with conforming, you feel the freedom to speak your truth with compassion, integrity, and respect for others. You need only look within. Your personal power path is waiting to be forged according only to what feels aligned, good, and right to you, not according to what is working for someone else.

Kristi's Power Enabler

Over time, you will find it easier to identify those aspects of your life that heighten your energy and bring you joy, and those aspects that lower your energy and bring you discomfort. It will seem right and natural to spend the majority of your time nurturing that which brings joy. Additionally, you will increasingly feel compelled to be of service to others—to give of yourself as you help others to live better lives. Along with fostering increasing levels of purposeful joy, this service to others will provide you with a strong sense of belonging and fulfillment. Over time, progress and transformation are inevitable as your life's intricate web of thoughts, emotions, beliefs, and actions coalesce, producing internal certainty, heightened energy vibrations, and a joy that can and will change your world for the better.

PART IV

What's Holding You Back?

"You must maintain unwavering faith that you can and will prevail in the end, regardless of the difficulties, and at the same time, have the discipline to confront the most brutal facts of your current reality, whatever they might be."
—Jim Collins

By now, you know that you cannot co-create your intended external life while your internal life is in turmoil. You must clear the way for your emerging spiritual awareness through inner work that addresses any negative or destructive energy that may be holding you back. You must overcome the ego, doubts, and fears that make you feel bad, create static, and prevent your soul-view–aligned desires from being made manifest.

Earthly physicality presents many pitfalls. This translates to myriad opportunities for static to interfere with the messages the spirit realm is sending you. Over time, the awareness and purpose that come from living in alignment with your inspired soul-view will enable you to mitigate this static. You'll begin to recognize when static has crept into your frequency. The key is having the awareness and actions to restore balance to your energy resonance right away.

The typical aspects of life that lower your vibrational frequency are at the same time presenting you with some of Earthly life's greatest challenges. As you Live with Certainty, you'll gain perspective on how to accept these challenges, lessen their impact, and use them for continued learning and development.

CHAPTER 20

Ego

*"Our status among others is not a burden, it is an illusion.
Vanity is our own mirror, a way we are seduced by what we want to see."*
—Noah benShea

I, ME, MY, MINE—we've been conditioned as a society to maximize everything connected to these pronouns. Most of the evil in the world emanates from allowing inflated states of ego, and the accompanying perception that we are not connected to our fellow humans, to have control. Let's be clear, however—ego in and of itself is not a bad or evil thing. Its primary desire is to defend and safeguard your fragile sense of self-worth. However, moving through life allowing your ego to be firmly in charge of your decisions and feelings is akin to being on board an airplane that's descending through a cloud layer. It's bumpy, turbulent, and you can't see anything past your nose no matter how hard you look out the window. So it goes with ego—ego is an illusion—and defining yourself according to an illusion is dysfunctional.

The fact is, however, that ego is an intrinsic part of human life. What we must do then is learn to effectively navigate life with it. Your genetics, conditioning, sense of security (or lack thereof), beliefs, and feelings all come together to create your ego. Ego has an unconscious effect on everything that you do, say, think, and feel. Your ego plays roles based on the labels you've assigned yourself. While this can bring you comfort, at times it can also wrap you up in a blanket of false security. When this happens, individuality and self-importance are taken too far, and you wind up elevating yourself above others.

Id, Ego, and Super-Ego

The famous psychoanalyst Sigmund Freud identified a structural model of the psyche comprised of three distinct parts: the id, ego, and super-ego. Freud maintained that the ego is the part of the mind which contains the consciousness. Initially, Freud used the word ego to refer to one's sense of self; however, he eventually modified this definition to refer to the mental functions of judgment, tolerance, reality-testing, control, planning, defense, intellectual functioning, and memory.

As defined by Freud, the id is a mass of instinctive drives and impulses, and demands immediate satisfaction. Like the mind of a newborn child, it has no sense of responsibility. It is amoral, illogical, and primarily sexual, and it won't take "no" for an answer. The super-ego is constantly watching every one of the ego's moves and punishes it with feelings of guilt, anxiety, and inferiority. To overcome this, the ego employs various defense mechanisms including denial, displacement, fantasy, compensation, projection, and rationalization. Because of their conflicting objectives, the super-ego tends to stand in opposition to the desires of the id, and is aggressive toward the ego.

Ego Isolates

A significant portion of the pain we experience in this world, and a great part of the pain that we inflict on others in our lives—even those whom we purportedly love—stems from our egos. Trying to control our lives so that we win and someone else loses is ultimately a source of great pain, envy, and frustration. Consider how much pain could be avoided if we didn't navigate the world as if it revolved only around us and our feelings; if we didn't feel offended or slighted at every turn. We spend an inordinate amount of time avoiding rejection, experiencing feelings of unworthiness, cultivating acceptance, attempting to control, questioning whether we are loved, and fearing the unknown. All of these states and efforts stem from the ego.

As a society, we have become self-absorbed and vain, consumed with doing things only for appearance's sake. The surface of life has overtaken the soul. It seems that our vanity, as opposed to authentic desire, controls what we do. We think that we're the most important person on the planet, and will do whatever it takes, even going so far as to hurt others, to make sure that we get what we want, do what we want, and don't experience anything that we don't want. When someone gets in our way, we're outraged. When we believe that our own happiness is the most important thing of all, and are willing do whatever it takes to achieve or maintain it, we only separate ourselves from our fellow humans.

Your ego is judgmental because it wants to defend and protect its self-image. It does this by criticizing others and diminishing anything or anyone critical of it. When the ego imagines or perceives any kind of a slight or an attack, the most common response is to retreat into full protection mode. The ego does not want to be accountable; it wants to blame, criticize, and impugn—whatever it takes to protect the fragile self. Some of the most common ways that your ego is responsible for your negative feelings emerge when you feel insulted or offended; feel inferior or lesser; are envious of what others have and you don't have; or are worried what people might be saying or thinking behind your back.

What Does an Unhealthy Ego Look Like?

We've established that the ego is the source of a lot of the destruction and negativity in the world, and that many of your most painful feelings are ultimately caused by your ego. The desires to win, to be right, and to experience pleasure and avoid pain are often primary reasons behind suffering. But if your current sense of yourself is the only one that you have ever known, how do you discern whether or not your ego is a problem? It's easier than you may think—but prepare yourself, because your Truth is likely going to be very different than your ego's view. Since your ego is not in touch with your soul's purpose, your sense of reality and security may be completely challenged as you discover your purposeful authenticity.

Stripping Your Ego of Its' Dominance

Your ego is the sum total of your thoughts and has everything to do with the way you define yourself: high-achiever, attorney, manager, mother, brother, author, college graduate, breadwinner, and so on. While you may describe yourself in a certain way and feel pretty good about your accomplishments, this is all ego-speak. It has nothing to do with living a life of purposeful authenticity and deep-soul joy. As hard as it may seem to let go of these ego-based identities, it is truly the only way to begin to live with certainty.

Your ego makes it difficult to maintain a consistent feeling of Source connectivity and unity. It is only as you become a removed, objective observer of your life that you begin to experience true awareness and become able to weaken your ego. First, you may need to undo years of conditioning, and banish a few misconceptions that have so far allowed your ego to dominate your thoughts and life. As you make progress in these areas, fragile and dysfunctional feelings of self-importance naturally fade away, and you become happier and more peaceful. One day, you'll suddenly realize that you no longer feel constantly hurt, insulted, or affronted by others. In the past, you may have experienced these feelings so often that you've been conditioned to believe that this is just how life is. While these voices are obstinate—even seemingly immovable—they can be banished. If you can't do this on your own, then it may become necessary to seek the help of a therapist. Remember, there is only strength and integrity in admitting that you need this help.

Stripping your ego of its dominance calls for gentleness, silence, stillness, meditation, and being willing to slow down. As you surrender to your feelings of pain and inadequacy, and permit yourself to experience them, you allow your inspired soul-view to strip the power from your ego. You begin to heal as you disengage your ego's stranglehold on your thoughts and feelings. Your ego deflates as you remove its coat of armor of conditioned, repressed responses. This is how you heighten your awareness, and how you create the space for your inspired soul-view to emerge.

The next time you are offended, step back from your thoughts and emotions. What's left? How do you feel deep inside? Once you get past your initial emotional responses, you may be surprised to learn that you feel fine. You'll realize that it wasn't a big deal after all. While it's very difficult to observe these events without becoming emotional in your reactions, Living with Certainty will help you. Through awareness, you'll start to reduce the ego's influence, and begin to live with authenticity, resiliency, and security—even during difficult and trying times.

Inspired Soul-View Versus Ego

Discovering your inspired soul-view is imperative to truly understanding that your various ego-personalities are not the real you. Any limiting, negative, critical thoughts, and voices in your head that want to compete, manipulate, overpower, or demean you aren't the authentic you. They emanate from your ego, not from your inspired soul-view.

Ego loses control as you awaken, become aligned with your inspired soul-view, and embrace universal interconnectivity—thereby expanding your world. Until you do this, your ego is the boss, and you are not co-creating the life the universe always intended for you to live. Your ego carries the power to make or break you, and it's only through awareness that you are able to begin seizing control from your ego and returning that power to where it should be—with your soul.

Embarking upon the journey to discover your truest self and purposeful authenticity takes an unwavering fearlessness, for your essence may be revealed as someone quite different than the ego-personality with whom you have always identified. If attempting to diminish your ego makes you feel as though you are losing a part of yourself, you are not.

With your ego in charge, there can be no real spiritual transformation. *Much* of the Living with Certainty approach is about supporting your efforts and hard work toward weakening your ego so that you can unearth your essence—your true self. You'll never experience a deep and intrinsic connection to Source energy and your fellow humans while your ego is allowed to be in charge. All of this takes courage, but take heart: Source energy is on your side. You are wired to do this.

Since the day you were born, your ego-personality has been conditioned to keep you agitated, turbulent, excited, mindless, attached to outcomes, virtually unaware, and completely out of alignment with your inspired soul-view. Your ego is the opposite of your essence, and can act as a hindrance or impediment to living with certainty. Your inspired soul-view, on the other hand, is steady, reliable, and always makes you feel good.

Once you live in alignment with your inspired soul-view, the ego no longer serves a purpose, and you will come to know yourself at a deep and authentic level. Once you understand what it feels like to live in alignment with your inspired soul-view, you'll become much more sensitive to the negative feelings that accompany your ego-personality any time that they emerge.

What Does a Healthy Ego Look Like?

When you live with certainty in all aspects of your life, you are living in balance with an authentic, healthy sense of self-confidence. Having a well-developed, healthy ego is a good thing. When you are joyous and enthusiastic about your life and who you are, there's no real advantage to being modest and self-deprecating. Here are some examples of how a healthy ego looks and feels.

- You view others more softly, through a lens of compassion.
- You are able to cope and find your way through the world.
- You share your enthusiasm with the world, but never at anyone else's expense or with the intent to harm or make anyone feel bad.
- You are humble, a sign of the truly self-confident.
- You encourage yourself and others.
- You spend time feeling good about your achievements, while giving thanks for your abilities, blessings, and opportunities.
- You spend time every day focusing on what is good and right in your life.

- You are endlessly grateful for every aspect of yourself and your life.
- You are naturally inclined to be of service to others because you sense your universal interconnectivity.
- You practice a balanced approach to your inner and outer life.

Your Ego and Living with Certainty

Exploring the ego is critical to Living with Certainty, for it's the only way to differentiate between the various voices in your head. You must move past the ego as part of your inner awakening process, even though your ego will want you to close off and surround yourself with walls, rather than venture into this new realm called Living with Certainty.

Don't think you have to rid yourself of your ego. The key is to keep your ego in balance by developing the awareness to know when your ego is preventing you from living with certainty, and has pulled you out of alignment with the flow of your spiritual power frequency. Any internal resistance you experience to living with certainty will emanate from your ego. It takes an unrelenting, conscious daily effort to subdue and overcome this negative, limiting voice. You'll know that your ego is in balance when you are able to live with certainty without willfully ignoring or violating any of the Energy Enablers, and you find yourself worrying less about what other people think and do. You needn't be perfect—we can all live with certainty while simultaneously celebrating our humanness.

One last thought—beware of your ego's voice in the spiritual process. If you start to feel inflated and self-righteous because you're following a spiritual path, you have not conquered your ego. If you would rather tell people you are following a spiritual path than to actually live with certainty, this is a strong sign that your ego is still in charge. The key at all times is to continue the plan, utilize the Energy Enablers, and keep growing.

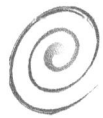

CHAPTER 21

Negative Thoughts

*"Life does not consist mainly—or even largely—of facts and happenings.
It consists mainly of the storm of thoughts that is
forever blowing through one's head."*
—Mark Twain

THOUGHTS ARE ILLUSORY and intangible. Despite this, they have the power to jerk you around like a Great Dane on a leash. Which of your thoughts seem to be on a continuous loop—old relationships, career regrets, bitterness toward others who may have wronged you? Thoughts serve to stoke the fires of past wrongs. As you undertake Living with Certainty, these unproductive thoughts must be eliminated. In all likelihood, they have been with you for years and have shaped your beliefs, feelings, actions, and circumstances.

The problem with this is that over time, you begin to self-identify with negative thoughts—particularly those that dwell on your past. You begin to think that you're the victim of this or that past circumstance or event, and then carry these feelings about yourself from your past into your future. When this happens, you can develop a very fragile sense of self. Negative self-talk can prolong and intensify the feelings of past wrongs, blowing them out of all proportion. Be aware that negative and self-defeating thoughts can completely prevent you from living with certainty.

Some people over-think, and some people just don't think at all. So often people say that they simply cannot control their thoughts. They let their thoughts run rampant, especially at night. This makes them feel terrible, and yet they claim that there's nothing they can do about it. This isn't true—healthy individuals can learn to control their thoughts. It is an issue of choice, will, and discipline. You simply have to take control and refuse to play the victim any longer. It is self-indulgent, undisciplined, and unwise to allow your thoughts to run amok. Thoughts needn't be reflexive, involuntary, or automatic. If they are, your mind and frequencies will become densely jammed with the resulting static.

Many, if not most, thoughts require no further action or air-time. Think of a thought as a feather blowing in a light breeze. As it floats by, it may seem suspended in mid-air momentarily, catching your attention before it's quickly blown away, never to be seen again. Notice your thoughts and then quickly push the self-defeating, non-soul-view–aligned ones out of your mind before they can create negative emotion and vibrate negative energy. Your goal is to create room for more positive, life-affirming thoughts.

Living with Certainty will help you to develop the ability to ensure that all thoughts are fleeting unless you *choose* for them to be otherwise. And, when you do need to spend some extra time contemplating and considering a significant matter, you do so objectively until the issue is resolved and/or you have a go-forward game plan. Then you move on. Be aware that there are times when persistent, unshakeable thoughts need to be addressed. Could it be your inspired soul-view guiding you to reconsider a decision or move in a certain direction? When an issue keeps cropping up, take note and deal with it until there's a resolution.

You may experience thoughts with no beginning or end. Your mind is ceaselessly cluttered with junk, and you must learn to control this mental chatter. This is most easily accomplished through silence, solitude, and awareness, and through developing your meditation practice. It takes effort to create an open space in your mind—but once you do, you'll see that it feels right. Over time, it will become second nature for you to still your mind when the chatter tries to take over.

You can also quiet your thoughts and bring peace to your life when you detach yourself from specific outcomes and expectations. This is accomplished by not allowing your thoughts to settle on any one right way. Stay open and have faith that events are being unfurled in a manner that will provide you with opportunities to learn and grow.

Negativity

Feeling down, blue, defeated, or stuck in the mud? Anxiety, worry, obsession, fear, and other emotions that feel bad begin with a negative thought, and remove you from the here and now moment. Research has shown that over-thinking is associated with many mental health disorders. The bottom line? Eliminate limiting, self-defeating thoughts—and, if necessary, seek help in eradicating them.

Negative thoughts create emotions that leave you feeling bad—anxious, angry, sad, remorseful, or lonely. They co-create experiences and circumstances for you that are likely the polar opposite of what you really want. The energy of these feelings is dense and low-vibrating. Goodness, consisting of fine, pure, high-vibrating energy, cannot be attracted by this dense, negative energy. As a matter of fact, the static inherent in this negative energy may very well deter everything good that you want to experience in your life, and even worse, attract everything that you *don't* want. A dense, low-vibrating frequency can only serve to make you feel awful, remove you from the flow of your spiritual power frequency, and reduce the likelihood that you will take soul-view–aligned action.

So how do you take control over these negative thoughts? With awareness, discipline, and fortitude you can learn to stop these thoughts from originating in the first place. The first step is becoming aware of how often you engage in negative thought so that you can begin to change the habit. Going forward, you have to embrace the mindset that you are a powerful creature of free will, and are fully in control of your inner experiences, including your thoughts. What you decide to co-create should be a deliberate choice.

It's precisely when times are the toughest that you have to summon every bit of awareness and fortitude within yourself, bolstering your vigilance not to allow negative thoughts and worst-case scenarios to fill your mind. Your most difficult challenge may involve successfully creating positive thoughts under demanding circumstances. You may find yourself experiencing tremendous sorrow or heartache due to circumstances beyond your control, yet you must not allow your thoughts to make things worse. Instead, make the choice to allow your thoughts to serve as a beacon bringing the hope, faith, and resilience needed to get you through tough times. Allow them to buoy you up, instead of pulling you farther down into the depths of despair.

Are Your Thoughts Truth?

How can you begin to diminish the feel-bad thoughts passing through your head every day, along with the subsequent negative effects they have on you? Start by accepting that just because you have a thought doesn't make it true; it may even be complete nonsense. You may well have tortured yourself believing things that aren't at all based in fact or truth. Your perceptions of your thoughts get whipped around based on a variety of factors: the level of guilt you have around the subject; how rested you are at the moment; how paranoid you are; what else you have going on in your life; past conditioning and beliefs; the amount of anxiety created; and many other reasons.

As thoughts appear, begin questioning their validity—don't automatically give weight or credence to them. Negative thoughts echo and reverberate around your mind, causing you to accept them as truth and to feel a whole host of negative emotions that torture you when, in fact, these thoughts aren't truth at all. Your brain can't tell the difference between truth and erroneous, negative mental chatter. You must not only learn to control your thoughts, but to disconnect from them.

A technique I once learned is to imagine a red stop sign appearing in your mind that replaces any negative thoughts that appear. Then make an appointment with yourself (say, 4:00–4:15 p.m. next Tuesday) to revisit this issue for a finite period of time.

Positive thoughts are aligned with your inspired soul-view and bring you closer to your soul mission, or your purposeful authenticity, through their pure, high-vibrational energies. They feel good, right, and purposeful. Your thought goal should be purity, purpose, and infinite goodness—no malice, no bias, no envy, no negativity, no "my way or the highway" (which are resultant states of your ego). When you create a positive thought, you've automatically transcended or risen above the dense smog to a finer vibratory level where you are more likely to co-create all of the wonderful aspects of your inspired soul-view. When you have a positive thought that feels good and purposeful, revel in it, think about it, and take it in.

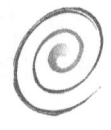

CHAPTER 22

Conditioning

"Man alone, of all the creatures of the earth, can change his own pattern. Man alone is the architect of his destiny."
—William James

YOU MAY HAVE DEVELOPED a lifetime of habits and conditioned thinking that are not at all in alignment with who you are. In fact, they may even be completely counter to the authentic you. Your soul-view has nothing to do with conditioning. You, along with your ego and all of the people, institutions, and circumstances that have influenced and surrounded you up until this point in your life's journey, have created a false identity for you. At some level, you may believe this is the real you. Your job now—and this will test you—is to free yourself from this artificial, surface identity and uncover and empower the soul-You that will guide the rest of your life.

Conditioning is essentially subconscious programming that directly affects how you view every aspect of your life. It's the result of beliefs passed on to you by an array of circumstances, outside forces, pressures, and influences. You have been conditioned throughout your life by thousands upon thousands of words, facial expressions, rules, limits, doctrines, and so on.

We are all impacted to various extents by the conditioning from society, media, schooling, peer pressure, language, early childhood experiences, relationships, socioeconomic conditions, and the like. Especially powerful forces include the beliefs and approaches to life held by our loved ones; the physical location in which we were born and raised; the things that we were taught were taboo to discuss; our

Chapter 22: Conditioning

family's secrets or lies; limits placed on us by family, educators, and religious leaders; and our parents' perceived success or failure in their own lives. These things have formed your subconscious beliefs and have conditioned you to think and believe as you do today. They have formed the basis for your values, beliefs, expectations, ideas, and perspectives.

Your conditioning unconsciously colors how you see the world—whether you are an optimist or a pessimist; whether you focus on light or dark; whether you have a fight or flight orientation to life; and so on. These perspectives can limit your belief in yourself, keep you stuck in the muck, and prevent you from developing and progressing. Further, it is a trap to identify yourself according to your memories and longings, since these things may not be relevant to your soul identity, which is the real you.

Children tend to begin life with natural authenticity, genuineness, and truthfulness. However, in our formative years we are like sponges as we observe the adults who surround us. As children, we have no defense mechanism to prevent us from accepting criticism and internalizing the beliefs of others. This conditioning changes children and their Source energy-given attitudes. Sadly, it is the people who raise us and surround us in our early life who rob us of so much belief, limitlessness, and confidence. Our caregiver's fears and dysfunction become our fears, mistrusts, dislikes, and shortcomings. These authority figures and influencers plant the seeds of our subconscious beliefs. If we tell children repeatedly that they are smart, they begin to believe they are smart. This enables them to approach the world thinking they are smart. As we reward and punish our children, we are conditioning them in a way that will impact them for their entire lives.

Humans tend to categorize life and its events into three buckets—things that we find agreeable and pleasurable, that which we find objectionable, and that which we really don't care about. Moving through life with these kinds of categorizations and judgments isn't healthy. Clearly, you must assess those things that can bring you danger and harm—but when applied universally to every aspect of your life, categorizations, labels, and judgments will limit your experience and possibilities. The goal is to escape this conditioning and instead learn to open your self while relying on your internal instruction system.

Your daily reactions to life are conditioned responses. If they're not working for you, you need to find a way out of these patterns so you can discover new, more authentic ways of responding to life. Escaping your early conditioning is difficult, but it is possible to change negative attitudes and conditioning.

Developing awareness is the first step toward undoing your conditioning. By becoming aware of those times when something triggers emotions or feelings, and then allowing yourself to experience those feelings, you open the door to healing. The more conscious thought you give to what triggers pain, the more you can diminish the intensity of these feelings over time. Experiencing painful feelings provides an opportunity to heal the root cause of the pain by uncovering your real wounds.

Through awareness, and by becoming increasingly sensitive to your energy, emotions, and instincts, you can reprogram your reactions and responses. As you become more aware of your energy, you can more easily change those habitual responses that are not truly in alignment with your inspired soul-view, or that don't allow you to vibrate energy at a pure, high-frequency. Make no mistake, identifying, recognizing, and shifting a life's worth of conditioning is hard work, but if you are to live with certainty, it's also essential and profoundly rewarding work.

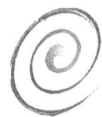

CHAPTER 23

Failure and Regret

"My imperfections and failures are as much a blessing from God as my successes and my talents, and I lay them both at his feet."
—Mohandas K. Gandhi

THERE IS NO SUCH THING AS FAILURE; there is only experience. The word failure is attached to ego. It is a label we place on efforts, events, and circumstances that don't work out as we had planned, hoped, or expected. Defeats, disappointments, and misses happen to everyone. Mistakes, bad choices, slip-ups, blunders, and oversights are all part of the process of living. We all experience failures. Our best laid plans can go out the window with one unanticipated turn of events—disease, accident, oversight, you name it. And no matter what happens, not trying or giving up is always far worse than failing.

Failure is feedback. Yes, it hurts (primarily our egos) when we fail, or our dreams are shattered and we experience depths of sorrow that we never thought were possible. But failure also stretches us beyond our comfort zone so that we may grow and develop our capacity to handle these events. Through failure, we are presented with some of our most significant learning opportunities. Ironically, we often profit more from the lessons learned and experiences gained through failure than if we had gotten what we had hoped for in the first place. The experiences of failure and suffering are pivotal aspects of personal development, through which we learn about our soft spots and how and when to change course. Every misfortune, every moment of despair, provides us with an opportunity to develop compassion and become more enlightened.

The key to accepting failure without allowing it to break you down is to embrace the fact that you were meant to experience whatever it is that you're going through. You needed this lesson in order to develop and move yourself on to the next level. Failure does not define you; it only develops you.

You must learn to bend and amend with failure. If you don't like an outcome, try again from this new place in which you now find yourself. The learning you gain from an outcome that you judge to be less than optimal gives you the perspective to try a new approach. One event closes, another appears on the horizon. Get back on your horse and ride. Winners and champions consistently fail, learn, and then contemplate their next move. Strength comes from believing that no matter what happens, you can survive and prevail. As hard as it may be to believe now, as you master the art of Living with Certainty, you will grow in your ability to experience a failure or setback more as an observer than as a participant.

Regret

You cannot allow regret to paralyze you. Feelings of regret prevent you from living in the here and now, while at the same time creating dense, negative, static-filled energy. Regret serves no productive purpose because it cannot solve a problem or undo a mistake.

As you live with certainty, you will rarely, if ever, experience regret again. The next time you start to wish you had handled something differently, shift your thoughts to this: *Thank you for providing me with better tools through such powerful development. I am so much better equipped now to deal with whatever comes my way.* This shift in your thought-focus away from regret and toward gratitude immediately allows you to clear up the static in your thoughts and heighten your vibrational frequency. As you find the silver lining, you will immediately feel better, remember your faith, and align with Source energy, which is constantly providing these experiences for your learning and personal development.

Regret does have its merits. It means that you're taking time for introspection and self-assessment. It can motivate you: *I don't ever want to feel that way again.* Allow yourself time to lament so you can feel and experience the mistake or loss. But give yourself no more than a few days to allow this feeling to pass. When time is up, you're done. After immersing yourself in your regret, the intense feelings will begin to lighten or wear away a bit. If you can't get over it, or if your load simply doesn't lighten, then contemplate what it is that you miss the most. What is the precise source of your pain, and how can you fill the void that has been left behind? You need to address the specific holes and emptiness you're feeling by adding opportunities and experiences that bring you new joy, fulfillment, and excitement. You need a win—something that will exponentially heighten your energy level.

They say hindsight is 20/20. That's true—it means we have learned the lesson. So learn and move on. You are now in another moment— the here and now. There's no point in wasting the present moment because of what happened in the past. Perhaps you are right, and you shouldn't have done whatever it is you did. But it *is* done, and it's way too late to change anything.

Accept that mistakes are an inevitable part of life. Living with regret is pointless. The time for thinking, planning, and listening to your internal instruction system was *before* you took the action you now regret. Once you've made the choice and taken the action, you have no choice as you live with certainty but to move on and look forward, not backward. You did the best you could; you did not intentionally try to fail. Shift your thought-focus to your soul-view and purposeful authenticity; over time your uncomfortable feelings about the past will begin to dissipate. You now see a better path, and you know a better way.

Moving Forward

Memories can be a great blessing, bringing you enormous joy as you relive wonderful events and moments from your past. However, when you obsess over negative memories by playing them over and over again in your mind in a destructive, recurring loop, they become a serious, life-altering problem. Going over the same old issues repeatedly is unhealthy physically, mentally, and spiritually. When your mind is stuck in the past, you stay tied to emotional baggage that prevents you from living with awareness of the here and now. Your past has left you with a load of worry and pain that encumbers you and weighs you down. You must break the habit and the conditioning of this destructive pattern through awareness and discipline. Filling your mind with negative events from the past is for victims, not powerful co-creators.

Wrong may have been done to you, which may not be "fair", but you must weigh justice versus continual punishment to your spirit. Not all things in life will be resolved to your satisfaction. Your power resides within you, and only you can determine how much power you will give to your transgressors. Take heart, though, because karma will win out where the perpetrator is concerned. In the toughest of cases, therapy may be warranted to facilitate your healing. Again, undergoing therapy in no way implies weakness. Quite the contrary, it shows strength, courage, and self-respect. You can derive great benefit from it. You must do whatever it takes to get your feelings out in the open. By acknowledging and experiencing them, you allow your feelings to dissipate in intensity, thereby providing yourself with relief. Whatever you do, do not dwell on these negative memories or feelings. You need to process them as quickly as possible and then lay them to rest.

Remember, whatever it is that has traumatized you is in the past. Now, you have two feet firmly planted in the here and now. Moving on doesn't diminish the wrong; it just means it's over and in the past. In the present of the here and now, you can be in control of your attitude and how you feel.

Whether you have known it before or not, you are empowered to begin creating the rest of your life's tale. This past event that has traumatized you will probably fall somewhere in the first or second act, but you certainly don't have to allow it to be the final one. Write a new script for your glorious next act and your grand finale. Pain need not be the end. Instead, you can allow it to create a new beginning.

If you waste time fighting the facts of the past, life will make Swiss cheese of you. Denial doesn't serve any useful purpose except to allow the past's negative baggage to create tomorrow's experiences. If you want to change your life, create new thoughts to serve as fuel for your new life. The past is over and done and has no power over you. So seize your power and take charge by grounding yourself firmly in the present, and by allowing yourself to take root in the here and now.

There is nothing standing in your way—the universe is not judging you. So, while you may be clinging to regrets, past failures, slights, affronts, and embarrassments, the creative energy plane is there waiting for you to let go of your negative thoughts, heighten your energy vibrations, and create anew in alignment with your inspired soul-view.

Blame and Resentment

Take personal responsibility for your every choice and decision and move beyond the need to blame others. Only victims lay blame. Do you really want to be a victim of your own life? As you blame others, point fingers, and feel resentment, you're making yourself and all those whom you're blaming feel worse, while keeping yourself living in a cloud of toxic dust. Until you cleanse these thoughts from your mind, your energy will be dense, low vibrating, and filled with static.

What are you hoping to achieve through blame? Does it really make you feel better by shifting the responsibility for your choices to someone else? The answer is no, not deeply or authentically. Blame and resentment are momentary crutches. Ultimately, resentment is toxic to your soul. Until you take responsibility for your actions, reactions, responses, choices, and experiences, you cannot move your life forward and into the light. You know the old saying—the best revenge is to live well.

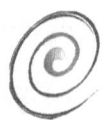

CHAPTER 24

Adversity and Problem Solving

"Each problem has hidden in it an opportunity so powerful that it literally dwarfs the problem. The greatest success stories were created by people who recognized a problem and turned it into an opportunity."
—Joseph Sugarman

LIFE IS MAGNIFICENT—it carries the power to inspire and enlighten us. But life also is miserable—it carries the power to break us down. This is the reality where we must find the balance, or center, from which we can live a Source energy–aligned life. Problems and conflicts are a major source of our pain and stress, and we can reduce their effect on us by altering our perception of them.

Every problem exists to rouse you, teach you vital lessons, and provide opportunities for learning and forward progress. Most problems appear out of nowhere, taking you from your inner world into a state of full awareness. When the rug gets pulled out from under you, your initial reaction most likely will be anxiety, anger, or fear. These feelings need to end quickly before they create detrimental static. In this respect, problems serve as catalysts. They rouse your true feelings, instincts, and compassion, allowing you to get in touch with what you really feel. They also come with a silver lining of lessons, course corrections, and growth opportunities—making them stepping stones that take you to a new level and a new place in your journey.

Living with Certainty requires that you take responsibility for your problems and their inherent lessons. As you open yourself to the lesson, you will cease blaming and falling into the same old conditioned, reactionary patterns. You'll no longer use problems as excuses for your failure to move forward. Shifting your thinking from seeing problems to instead seeing opportunities can propel you to the next level.

You will bring yourself immense peace if you cease to identify, label, and judge circumstances as good or bad. Instead, accept what is, take stock of how you feel, and look for the lesson. With your goal to live with certainty and live as static-free as possible, you become more thoughtful and less reactionary; you stop focusing as much on the conflict and spend far more time on resolution and doing the right thing. You take comfort in the fact that you're not alone in your decisions or choices. You know that a higher power is working with you through your intuition, internal instruction system, and your inherent creative ability to help you solve your own problems.

Focusing on and envisioning an effective solution or end-result raises your vibrational frequency energy and makes you feel good. The best responses and solutions will resonate with you because they feel good and right.

Problem Solving, Making Decisions, and Finding Solutions

Studies have shown that people who effectively handle stress have advanced coping skills that allow them to willingly assume control of their lives, live healthy lives that include exercise and relaxation, have significant relationships, enjoy humor, and espouse spirituality as an important aspect of their lives.[23]

You must remain proactive in the leadership of your life when adversity hits. It is your pain—and your desire for it to end—that will ultimately motivate you to change. Problem solving requires objectivity. You can't make a sound decision until you acknowledge reality. The trick here is that not everyone is willing to admit to themselves the reality of the situation and the real mess they may be in. Your ego kicks into overdrive in situations where you may actually be the culprit of the difficulty. As painful as it may be, and as resistant as your mind may be to admitting wrongdoing, muster the internal fortitude to admit your mistakes and deal with the facts. This is essential if you really want to make a good decision and remedy the situation. You have to clear your mind of the emotion, pain, and stress within that you have allowed the situation to create. Only when your mind is truly clear can you begin the process of accurate assessment. Retreat to stillness if needed to quiet the voices in your head that are discoursing in direct opposition to reality.

Problems must not be solved from a state of fear or denial. Rather, you must decelerate to a place of peace and clarity; solutions emanate more naturally from this state. All too often we fuel our problems and fan the flames by fretting, worrying, and obsessing over worst-case scenarios. By doing so, you are giving energy to exactly that which you do not want. Focusing on your problem in a manner that limits solutions and projects into worst-case scenarios only allows anxiety to build up, and makes your energy dense and low vibrating. If you focus on the scenarios that you don't want, you increase the likelihood that they will be made manifest. Your best bet is to jettison negativity. Become proficient at catching yourself beginning to spin your negative tales, and immediately transition your thoughts to that which you *do* want. Don't give more than a couple of seconds of thought to worst-case scenarios. Further, don't incessantly talk about your problems—only share them with your inner circle or those whose advice, ideas, and feedback you are seeking.

Living with Certainty requires that you learn to manage your problems in such a way that you maintain a high-frequency vibrational level. Stop telling yourself that you don't know what to do, or don't have the answer, and instead tell yourself that you're certain that you will come up with the answer. Believing that you are capable of coming up with the solution gets you focused and confident. Think deeply, and become aware of your feelings. What options tighten your chest and burden your solar plexus? What options open you up, make you feel better, relaxed, and bring a feeling of calmness and peace? Remember that problems are relative. Irrespective of what you are facing, someone else at some time has faced the same problem, and allowed him or herself to be defeated. Conversely, someone else has faced the identical problem—but chose to persevere and be creative, and triumphed magnificently, overcoming all that you now face. You are linked to that success story through universal interconnectivity. Allow that energy to inspire and embolden you.

CHAPTER 25

Criticism

"Be who you are and say what you feel because those who mind don't matter and those who matter don't mind."
—Dr. Seuss

WHAT OTHER PEOPLE THINK of you should be of no real consequence. A natural extension of living with purposeful authenticity is to stop craving the approval of others, or being overly aware of and concerned with their scrutiny. When you alter your deepest desires due to the opinions of and pressures from others, or out of a concern for social acceptance, you have forfeited living with certainty and are no longer maintaining the appropriate level of respect for your spiritual journey.

Criticism and Opinions of Others

As you spend time contemplating—even brooding over—how others perceive you, you are forming the basis for how you see yourself. You are letting others—even complete strangers—form your opinion about yourself and the value you bring to the world. If you find yourself routinely caught up in how you are perceived by others and are accustomed to seeking the approval of others, you have to break free of this cycle and dependency. This is a sure sign that your ego and vanity issues are significant.

Part of the reason that your inspired soul-view is hidden and muted today may be because you have given too much power to others, who then projected their labels, beliefs, and hopes for you onto you. Being the people-pleaser you are, you internalized these opinions. You can never forfeit your personal power, authenticity, and freedom in order to conform to the desires or demands of others. When you do so, you lack courage and self-assurance, and have placed being approved of and liked above everything that really matters.

Constructive Criticism

We receive more "constructive" criticism from people than we really want or need. Sure, some of it helps us to grow and develop, and as you live with certainty, you'll become increasingly better at discerning those times when the opinions of others matter and when they don't. You must always remain receptive to counsel, guidance, and recommendations, but you should weigh this external feedback and information with respect to how it aligns with your inspired soul-view and internal instruction system. Learn from constructive feedback and criticisms where you can, but forget about receiving approval. Not only can you not please everyone, but you do not have to. Yes, living in harmony and peace with everyone is ideal, but it's not always realistic. You needn't build consensus or take a vote about how to live your life. True-life transformation comes about as you listen to and live in alignment with your inspired soul-view, not with the opinions and perspectives of others.

Listen to people you respect and hold in high regard. Seek their advice when needed and take it to heart. Certainly, part of living with certainty is to remain open, polite, and considerate, especially when faced with the opinions of others. But be balanced in how you process this information. Maybe there's a kernel of truth in what they're saying from which you can learn, but maybe there's not. Criticism from others is information—really nothing more than opinion. Other people are entitled to relay facts to you about a situation or event that needs to be discussed (and you are entitled to do the same).

A thick skin will serve you well. As difficult as it is, you have to muster the inner strength to deflect and not personalize others' negativity. Criticism and rejection are part of life. Just remember, all of the people in your life are human—flawed, wonderful, but human.

Many of them make themselves feel valuable by asserting themselves. It is well within your right to take their criticism or leave it. But if you take it, take it and learn from it. If you leave it because you see no value in it, then leave it. Don't stew over it or incessantly focus on your outrage or how offended you feel.

Keep Your Perspective When Egos Talk

When you find yourself getting the brunt of another's criticisms, know that their ego is talking, not their soul. You have created in them a desire to exercise superiority over you. This is one of those times that you must choose to live with certainty. Open your perspective, go to that peaceful place in your heart, and choose to not have a reaction. Remember, this critical commentary is coming from someone who has emanated from the same goodness as you—you are universally interconnected. Your goal must be to see beyond these comments and try to relate to the soul, not the ego, with whom you're interacting. Abusive, critical people are treating you in accordance with how they feel about themselves and their place in the world. Do you really want to place that much weight on the viewpoint of someone who is less than enlightened? As my husband's grandfather used to say, "If a jerk calls you a jerk, are you going to believe him?"

When you feel under attack and criticized—as if someone else is attempting to edit and censure your thoughts—your energy is in a serious state of discord, and you likely feel tense and incompatible with your inspired soul-view. Respectfully let these people know that you will take their viewpoint into account, and then exit this situation immediately so that you can once again clear and heighten your energy.

Aligning with Your Internal Instruction System Is What Matters

Knowing yourself is the only way to seize the power you possess to co-create your life. Your discovery of your inspired soul-view and your experience of deep-soul joy don't depend upon anyone else.

Naysayers are merely testing your level of commitment. If there is no semblance of truth in what someone is saying to you or trying to convince you of, if nothing is resonating positively, honor your internal instruction system, and hold true to your purposeful authenticity.

Self-Consciousness

Self-consciousness is a self-limiting feeling that occurs when you are more concerned about how others are observing and judging you than anything else. Your goal is to be self-aware, but not self-conscious. Other people will always think different thoughts than you, have different perspectives than you, and make different choices than you—*and that's fine.* They need to choose in alignment with their own internal instruction system, which will never be the same as yours.

Train your mind not to allow yourself to spend one minute of thought on how others perceive or judge your inspired soul-view-aligned actions. Think of the hurtful opinions of others as static—while you can learn from and appreciate some of it, some of it is simply white noise that can be disregarded. Know this, however—if you are concerned about how someone thinks about you, it's usually because you are feeling that way about yourself.

How others relate to you is largely a result of what you've taught them about how they can or should relate to you. Your relationships, the ones you wish to maintain, will go through a transition as you live with certainty. For example, if you have a history of asking for people's opinions, perhaps you'll continue to do so, but you also may choose to do so with less frequency or not at all as you focus on listening to your internal instruction system. If your patterns in this regard change, people will need to understand that you are now living with certainty and no longer wish to be bombarded with their unsolicited opinions.

Judging Others

You cannot live with certainty while judging people. Source energy does not judge—and it is your job to live your life in such a way that you emulate the high-vibrational, compassionate purity of Source energy as closely as you can. You must control judgmental thoughts because they hurt you by lowering your vibrational frequency. As you learn to accept and love yourself, you will find that you judge others far less.

You may have developed the habit of judging others to ease your fears about people and situations, to make yourself more comfortable, or to put things in a less-threatening perspective. Judgment is your ego's way of feeling better about itself. Labeling, categorizing, classifying, or characterizing others is wrong. Backgrounds or beliefs different than yours are not to be judged. This includes what people have, what they look like, what they sound like, what they do for a living, and so on. Everyone has different levels of ambition, but one is not superior to the other.

Certainly you must learn to be *discerning* and take note of people and circumstances that do not feel good or right. However, you can observe and acknowledge someone's behavior without attaching labels that carry emotion, judgment, or feelings of superiority. Remember that everything that appears in your life is there for a reason.

Be curious and kind, but not judgmental. If you want to soften your perceptions and judgments, imagine that the person you are judging is a family member—your brother, sister, mother, father, grandmother, or grandfather. Suddenly, patience and compassion come much easier.

Similarly, bias and prejudice have no place in living with certainty. Through the habitual act of judging others, you are creating negative energy and removing yourself from your spiritual power frequency. The soul does not judge, only the ego-personality judges.

You have no idea what is right for others, what they are meant to learn, what they should do, or what specific circumstances their souls are meant to experience. You must honor other's boundaries, choices, and limits if you want anyone to value your own.

Why We Judge

When you gossip, pass judgment, or spread negativity about others, you demonstrate that you don't feel very good about an aspect of yourself. When you judge others, you are making the mistaken assumption that you come from a place of superiority and moral high ground. You are never justified in your feelings of self-righteousness and resentment.

Why are we so aggravated and provoked by certain people? Usually it's because we see in them the qualities we dislike in ourselves—the very things that lower our energy and prevent us from living with certainty. These reactions are about us, not them.

If you are to stop judging others, you must first cease judging yourself. It is usually when you are not feeling good about yourself that you lash out at others. Begin the journey by becoming calmer, lighter, and gentler. Find something positive to think about those whom you've previously judged. If you can't do this, you must take a look at yourself. Are you unduly hard on yourself as well? Remember that when you look at others critically, you are going to attract more of that critical negativity into your own experience.

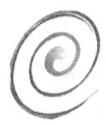

CHAPTER 26

Measuring Up

"There is a time in every man's education when he arrives at the conviction that envy is ignorance; that imitation is suicide; that he must take himself for better, for worse, as his portion."
—Ralph Waldo Emerson

IF YOU HAVE LED a life of comparison, competition, envy, and jealousy, it will be powerful and freeing for you to experience the way this negativity falls away as you naturally begin to experience the contentment and confidence that comes with living a life of purposeful authenticity. Once you uncover your inspired soul-view, self-love comes more easily, and the notion of comparing yourself to others seems increasingly absurd and trivial.

Envy, jealousy, competition, and comparison exist only in your mind thanks to your ego, which likes to isolate itself this way. As you live with certainty, however, you increasingly accept that while we are all connected at the level of essence, there is no value in comparing your life, success, and achievements with others. By virtue of our universal interconnectivity, we need and will be aided by others, but we are never to measure ourselves against our fellow humans. Rather, our benchmark should be how closely we emulate the vibrational level of Source energy through our everyday thoughts, beliefs, actions, and gratitude.

Without question, some people have suffered more hardship than others. While this isn't fair, we must understand that there is no concept of fairness in the ways of our universe. There are only our intended lessons.

Let go of the lack of fairness you've been focused on and replace it with a more productive thought focus. A so called lack of fairness may have caused you to endure the very hardships that have prepared and strengthened you for the next level of your Earthly experience. This isn't to say that suffering is by its very nature good. Clearly no one wants to endure it. But what doesn't kill you makes you stronger through teaching you invaluable lessons.

Congratulate and Wish Others Well

Give due congratulations, accolades, recognition, and kudos to others, even when this direct "competition" in your mind has won a battle and you're not happy about the outcome. When you do this, you shift the frequency of your energy level to one far more positive and life affirming.

All too often, we attempt to slander and disempower our competitors, but if we could just remember that we're all interconnected souls, we would choose to behave differently. Competition is clearly a man-made concept; the truth is that there is nothing but unlimited abundance in the world. If we could truly understand this, we would not harbor such negative, self-defeating, and distracting feelings.

Embrace Your Own Gifts

When you don't have a sense of the authentic you, you can become severely lacking in confidence and self-assurance. As you discover your inspired soul-view, however, you know that your success and the abundance available to you aren't based on what anyone else has or does. There is no need to compete. We are all unique, different, and diverse, and we should like it that way. The universe benefits from this diversity.

Regardless of who you compare yourself with, you will have the same life—you'll be just a bit more miserable. If you compare yourself to people who have either more or less, you may feel either good or bad. As you resent the success of others, you emit negative energy, thereby harming your own life experience and weakening your ability to co-create. Instead, celebrate the success of others if you want to see more success in your own life. Extend love to others and begin focusing on expressing your own purposeful authenticity and joy.

Jealousy

Feelings of jealousy are creatures of your own mind, and are detrimental and destructive to your personal energy. Allow your heightened awareness and internal instruction system to alert you to feelings of jealousy so that you may quickly shift to a more positive, comforting mindset. Otherwise, these feelings may draw more obstacles and competition into your life. The silver lining of jealousy is that it exists to make you aware of your own need to heal some of your own shortcomings and soft spots.

Competition

Competition stems from the fear that you will not measure up, will be revealed to be a failure, or will look bad due to someone else's success. You worry that there won't be enough for you. Once again, you can thank your ego for your feelings of inferiority to those who somehow, in your mind, have more than you.

Businesses and corporations must compete effectively in order to survive and thrive. However, the competition that exists between individuals is the natural outgrowth of our external search to fill internal voids. At the root of this interpersonal competition lies the desire for power—and this is the root of much conflict and hate in the world. As social beings, most of us live and work in communities filled with other unfulfilled humans. This will never lead to strong, compassionate human relations. We must change.

When you're living competitively, you haven't found your own way yet; you aren't living in alignment with your inspired soul-view. Living with a scarcity mindset causes you to feel as if we all are competing for a limited supply of material and professional success, power, and accomplishment. Once you understand, however, that it is unnecessary to compete with anyone for anything, you begin to realize how much time and mental energy you've poured into the wrong things. Yes, some people will always have more than you, and you, in turn, will always have more than others. This is inevitable, since we're all unique individuals with unique souls living unique lives. Rather than spending time competing with others, use that time to live with certainty so that you can exploit your own unique potential for the rest of your life.

Focus on abundance. Any time you feel territorial and competitive, you're focusing on a *lack* of something, rather than on the *creation* of what you want. There are unlimited supplies of everything and anything good in the universe—more than enough for everyone. It is people who feel alone and inferior who focus the most on competition. You're not battling the world; you're not competing for finite amounts of anything. You are an empowered co-creator.

Comparison

You are a unique individual in a unique place and time in the universe. Be authentic—bring forth your own unique experiences, emotions, passions, and personality, and let go of imitation. When you are consumed with measuring up, you lose your focus and your authentic ability to create. Everyone's life is intended to be different. We each have our own strong points and special gifts. Don't allow thoughts of comparison to others to ever enter your mind.

When you find yourself feeling competitive or comparing yourself to others, stop. Remind yourself that these very thoughts will stymie all of your other efforts to discover your deep-soul joy. Don't allow this weakness of imitation, comparison, and competition to take you off track. Over your lifetime, you have developed your own gifts in a unique way. Use them and seize the opportunities with which they present you.

Abundance

One of the overarching concepts of this book is that we live in an abundant universe. We all have the potential to experience an abundance of joy, love, learning, freedom, self-actualization, money, compassion, and other wonderful things. Modern society creates within many of us a pressure to strive for the Mercedes, mansion, and big bank account. But these material pleasures are not a requirement for experiencing the most profound levels of deep-soul joy.

Abundance is an intrinsic part of our infinitely creative universe. It isn't necessary for others to have less—or to lose—in order for there to be enough for you. More for someone else does not mean less for you. You short-circuit the creation of your own abundance when you expend mental energy on thoughts of competition or taking away from others. Instead, by thanking the universe for its gracious abundance, you will attract more abundance into your experience. By helping others to achieve more, you actually create more for yourself.

Think in terms of limitlessness—no boundaries—as you place your thought-focus on creating a life in expression of your purposeful authenticity. Don't limit what you believe is possible for yourself to aspects of your life that already exist. As you create in alignment with your purposeful authenticity, follow the path of your passions, inspirations, and creativity. Allow these soul-inspired aspects of yourself to lead you to discover unknown places and create anew.

CHAPTER 27

Forgiveness

"To be wronged is nothing unless you continue to remember it."
—Confucius

TO FORGIVE IS TO PARDON and renounce your anger or resentment against someone for a fault or offense they have committed. In other words, after spending time ruminating about how you have been wronged (initially a sign of a healthy self-respect), you make a choice to let go of the desire to punish by detaching yourself from all the baggage and negativity to which you've been clinging. Forgiving is releasing the negative in order to immerse yourself in the positive, which cannot be achieved as long as you are attached to an anchor of past wrongs and negativity. It provides emotional relief that sets you free from the shackles of umbrage and bitterness.

Forgiveness is about you, not the perpetrator. When you forgive, you are not excusing, condoning, or overlooking the actions of others. Rather, you make the decision to forgive for *yourself*, out of love for *yourself*. You make a decision to let go so that *you* can go on. It is possible that people who wrong you may not even care whether you have forgiven them or not. You do this for you, so that the person who has already hurt you once cannot prevent you from flourishing any longer. Forgiveness turns out to be your very best revenge because it heals and purifies *you* and *your energy*, enabling you to once again achieve a high vibrational frequency.

You can either remain closed, angry, fearful, and stuck in your pain, or you can open yourself, let go of the past, and forgive in order to move forward in your own life. You cannot live with certainty when you vibrate energy filled with a negative charge such as bitterness. Living a life of love and peace is impossible without forgiveness.

Why is forgiveness such an essential aspect of your spiritual journey? Because through forgiveness you align your own energy with Source energy, which provides you with the strength and fortitude to move forward without pain, feeling lighter, happier, and better about yourself. Living in alignment with Source energy enables you to live a life of grace which streams to you from the Source. It must, in turn, be extended from you to all others. To forgive is simply to open your heart to grace and a life of love—for yourself, for others, and for Source energy.

Forgiveness Is a Process

Forgiveness is true transformation, and it can feel extremely uncomfortable. You are forced to acknowledge and experience your hurt feelings rather than suppressing them any longer. Forgiveness takes empathy, guts, and a willingness to work through and endure some pain. A therapist may be invaluable as you work through your feelings and consider other perspectives. You have to put yourself in the offender's shoes if you are to gain perspective into his or her behavior. This is also the time to rely on the comfort of your meditation practice, deep-breathing techniques, and exercise (particularly exercise that simultaneously allows you to experience nature, such as outdoor walking, hiking, running, or cycling). All these techniques will help you reduce and deal with your stress. As the negative emotion subsides, you will be able to view the situation far more rationally and objectively.

Without a doubt, forgiveness is a process—something you will work on every day until the anger, resentment, and memories run their course and begin to fade. It forces you to be bigger than perhaps you ever thought possible.

Benefits of Forgiveness

Studies have shown that the physical benefits you enjoy as you release your anger and forgive are numerous, including lower pain and stress levels, reduction in blood pressure, and reduced incidences of general illness.[24]

You may think certain people don't deserve your forgiveness. That is not the point, since they may never even know whether you have forgiven them or not. Forgiveness is a personal, internal event that enables your own freedom while heightening your personal vibrational level. It is a gift you give to yourself out of respect for yourself. It releases you from the past and sets you free from negative thoughts. As the physical manifestations of stress, pain, and anxiety lessen throughout your body, it feels like your heart is opening. And *it is*. Forgiveness gives you a fresh start by healing your heart, soul, body, and thoughts. Once you experience this relief, you will understand why you must continue to let go.

Why We Can't Forgive

Forgiving those who have wronged us takes commitment and repeated attempts. Be patient and kind with yourself. Don't force it. If you find yourself at your core refusing to go along with the notion of forgiveness, you aren't ready. You have more internal work to do. Much of the inability to forgive comes from a desire to be vindicated. Holding out and refusing to forgive isn't going to change what has happened—it just prolongs the pain. And it will completely prevent you from developing and moving your life forward through living with certainty.

How Lack of Forgiveness Hurts You

An inability to forgive points to old, unhealed wounds. Releasing yourself from the pain of the past is difficult. As you choose to continue to give life to these feelings, you are injecting a daily dose of negativity into the here and now. This is unnecessarily tragic because you will never have the opportunity to live the life the universe always intended for you to live. When you bear a grudge and resent those who have wronged you, keep in mind the static you are creating in your own vibrational frequency. You are effectively allowing the perpetrator to play a further role in harming you in the here and now.

Blame

Blame doesn't enable you to feel better either. It's simply your justification for lacking the courage to experience and work through your pain. You may mistakenly believe that the only path to happiness is to continue to blame and condemn others. However, living with certainty requires that you abandon blame and resentment. And don't even think about revenge. Have faith that karma will take care of injustice. Life is short enough as it is. Don't give more of your present or your future to someone or something that has taken from you in the past.

Make a Choice to Forgive

With forgiveness, you make the decision to no longer carry the burden of resentment toward someone. Once you make this decision to forgive, every subsequent day you'll face the *choice* of not allowing negative thoughts to seep into your mind. As you make new choices about what you think and feel, you'll become increasingly empowered and allow yourself the freedom to finally live the life the universe always intended for you to live. Forgiveness is not denial. Nor is it about someone else winning and you losing. It is a mechanism for releasing the grasp of the past. Forgiveness is a way forward that releases the weight of things that cannot be undone.

Some days, the decision to forgive is harder than others, and the only way you can forgive is to view the perpetrator as a soul, perhaps tortured, but nevertheless a soul to which you are interconnected. You acknowledge that your souls both emanated from Source energy. You will forgive knowing it is not worth sacrificing your own spiritual journey for this undeveloped soul. By no means must you agree with what someone did in order to forgive them. Rather, you acknowledge the Earthly weakness, faults, and frailty of this person, and choose to forgive them for it. Remember, you are doing this for yourself—and your loved ones.

CHAPTER 28

Doubt

"Doubt whom you will, but never yourself."
—Bovee

TO HAVE DOUBT is to be undecided, skeptical, disbelieving, or distrusting. Doubt is a sign that you're not ready to make a decision. It's also a sign that you're not in an optimal situation. Doubt is an aspect of your internal instruction system intended to prevent you from making wrong choices and decisions. It makes no sense to move forward when doubt is present; the anchor of doubt will lower your vibrational frequency and weigh you down until you change course and rectify the situation. Any time you are filled with doubt prior to a decision, don't move in the direction you are considering, and don't make a decision until you consider alternatives that allow the feeling of doubt to dissipate.

While doubt will always serve as part of your internal instruction system, you are not living with certainty when you are frequently riddled with doubt. The surest way to experience less doubt in your life is to live in alignment with your purposeful authenticity and remain aware at all times of how you're feeling at decision time. In this way, you can rest assured that you're making the best decision possible at that moment.

CHAPTER 29

Denial

"To regret one's own experiences is to arrest one's own development. To deny one's own experiences is to put a lie into the lips of one's life. It is no less than a denial of the soul."
—Oscar Wilde

WHEN WE DENY SOMETHING, we are using a deeply ingrained defense mechanism to assert that something alleged is not true or to refuse to accept or believe something. If denial is a part of your current toolkit with respect to how you view yourself, it will stand in the way of your spiritual journey to live with truth. Denial is often accompanied by aggression—both are part and parcel of the victim mindset.

If you routinely become defensive, rejecting and rebuffing input and feedback from others while asserting that *it's not your fault,* you do indeed live with denial. If you dodge attempts by others to hold you accountable through the use of excuses, your denial habit is sabotaging your life. When you won't accept responsibility and never apologize, it negatively affects your energy and relationships. People will understandably grow hostile toward you since denying the truth is tantamount to lying. You are enveloping yourself in dense, low-vibrating energy and static. Nothing good that emanates from the creative energy plane can manifest through your thoughts when you live from a place of denial and disavowment.

If you find that you have a propensity for denial, spend time telling yourself that no one is perfect. You may be operating from a place of very low self-esteem, convinced that everyone else is better or more perfect than you. Not true. Everyone is flawed, and everyone has the potential for greatness and abundance, but only when we open ourselves, admit to our flaws or misdeeds, and do the necessary inner work to heal. The strongest, most vibrant people I know readily admit—usually with great humor—that they are far from perfect.

CHAPTER 30

Skeptics

"There are no atheists in foxholes."
—Unknown

AS DEEPAK CHOPRA HAS SAID, the simple fact is that whether you believe or not, the universe still goes on in its spiritual splendor, for it doesn't require your permission to work as it does. The laws of the universe are not dependent upon your approval. Whether you believe in a Higher Order or not, you are still a part of the intricate web of energy and spirit in which believers and non-believers all participate. Some skeptics act as if spirituality, superstition, and witchcraft are all the same. And some areas of science actively attempt to discredit the spiritual realm.

We are not living with certainty when we disrespect the beliefs of others through attempts to belittle, change or reform them. If we're all guided toward the end goal of deep-soul joy, let us not judge one another on how or whether or not we get there. Above all, have compassion for believers and non-believers alike.

The fact is that some people innately live with certainty—even atheists. This is possible because through living with certainty, you align your energy with Source energy—whether you believe in the existence of this alternate dimension or not. I once knew a skeptic who without a doubt lived with certainty. She was brilliant, passionate, and lived a life that expressed her purposeful authenticity. Her work was an extension of her natural abilities and inclinations and her success further fueled her drive and goals. She was fulfilled and extremely

Chapter 30: Skeptics

discriminating in how she spent her time and with whom she spent it. She communed with nature and lived with the highest integrity. She was surrounded by people whom she loved and whom, in return, adored her. She was completely and intrinsically connected to her inspired soul-view and Source energy—and yet she was in complete denial of the existence of Source energy.

Did she ever give thanks for this gifted life? I don't know. My guess is that in her own way, she did so every day until she became elderly and weak. Then she seemed miserable, floundering, purposeless, and mentally ready to die, even though her physical body wasn't ready. She had no faith to cling to, no hope that her soul would go on, no inner spiritual life whatsoever. Over the years, I have witnessed the old age of many family members, both atheists and believers alike, and there is no comparison between the fulfillment and peace experienced by the believers in their final days versus the non-believers.

Skeptics have been conditioned to be skeptical. This is a learned approach to life. We don't begin our lives as skeptics. Certainly, some level of skepticism is good as it causes us to examine and question our Truth and what we really believe. However, some skeptics tend to lord their self-perceived intellect over you. While we are all entitled to our own opinion, having a closed mind is not a good or enlightened way to live. Even if your inclination is to be skeptical, it is a far healthier and more intellectual approach to be *skeptically open*. None of us has 100 percent proof, but many of us have 100 percent faith and can point to experiential evidence.

Irrespective of what you believe, it is your responsibility to peacefully coexist with believers and non-believers and to fully allow everyone to believe in and express their own views. Anytime we begin to judge and make fun of another, we cross the line, lower our own energy vibrations, and reveal much about ourselves.

Don't feel that you have to justify your beliefs to anyone, or that you have to be practical or conservative in your beliefs. Anyone who attempts to force his or her beliefs or non-beliefs on you, particularly in a demeaning manner, is not living with certainty.

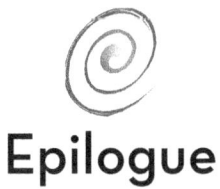

Epilogue

"It's never too late to be what you might have been."
—George Eliot

OUR PLANET IS IN CRISIS, and it needs our spiritual attention in a multitude of ways. Across the globe, we are steadily witnessing the worst of human behavior. This behavior is all too often deeply rooted in an ego-driven self-righteousness that has at its foundation an unmitigated separation of self from our souls, our fellow humans, nature, and the interconnected commonality of Source energy. This separation is destroying our planet, and the proof is in the distressing, man-made issues we presently face—war, famine, suppression, genocide, terrorism, human trafficking, and so on.

While this is a global issue, American culture in particular is rapidly becoming increasingly characterized by faded morals, a lack of graciousness, growing individuality, and selfishness. Many of us are exposed to these behaviors every day through our interactions with others. To make matters worse, we recognize these behaviors in *ourselves*. But we've also reached a point where we're willing to consider what we can do differently, because we don't like who we have become and how we feel. What if we could feel better? What if this spiritual energy that we increasingly sense is real and is being left untapped? What if we can seize the moment to be co-creators of something different than we've experienced to date? What if we stopped resisting our instincts telling us how powerful we are, and as a result of this enhanced focus and belief were authentically and profoundly able to expand and improve our lives?

Our fast-paced society with its outward focus and misplaced values has produced fleeting, media-induced dreams and desires driven by external stimulus rather than internal certainty. The invasiveness of the media and the ubiquitous access that many of us have to it has in part contributed to the soullessness we experience today. We are constantly bombarded by unnecessary, misleading, and often biased information and images that crowd our minds, leaving no room for the contemplation of what really matters. Sadly, many people no longer even know how to identify for themselves the things that really matter.

Now is the time to become aware of how you've been constructing your own blockages and impediments. This discontent emanating from a place deep within you is letting you know that you're not living true to yourself—your Earthly life is not what it should be; you are not living the life the universe intended for you to live. The fact that you haven't taken action up until now points to roadblocks. Maybe you are skeptical that a spiritual realm actually exists. Maybe you are fearful because you do believe in another dimension, but you have no idea what it means, where it is, or how to find it. Maybe you are surrounded by skeptics and are feeling embarrassed about exploring your spirituality for fear of ridicule. Maybe you need to heal and recover from a lifetime of bad mental habits and conditioning. Maybe the rigors of your daily life simply moved you away from your spiritual center, and you now need to return and re-examine your spiritual beliefs and practices.

Let's face it; our individual thoughts, beliefs, emotions, and actions have collectively created the mess we're in. The silver lining is that this upheaval has caused many of us to take the time to consider the workings of the universe, and to go deep within ourselves to find comfort and solace in an inner place of security and tranquility. All the while our instinct is signaling to us that from this place we can change and co-create a new world. Now is the time to utilize and leverage this knowledge about our ability to co-create our lives so that we not only improve our own circumstances, but also positively alter the current crash and burn trajectory of our planet.

Shakespeare's King Henry V said, "All things are ready if our minds be so." The time has always been right for as many of us as possible to come together and to connect under a fresh spirituality. In so many ways, the world and our lives are unpredictable and unstable. We worry about ourselves and about the world around us. For many of us, peace of mind has been replaced by anxiety, fear, and desperation; and our mental and physical health is suffering. While we cannot completely circumvent pain, we can control our reaction to it, and how deeply it affects us. We can learn from it, allowing it to make us better, stronger, more compassionate, and more purposeful. Take control of your spiritual and emotional life. It is the time to live with certainty.

All man-made problems that exist on the planet are *our* problems, not someone else's. We own them as much as anyone else. For far too long we have all pointed fingers, blamed others—and worst of all, we've looked the other way. Underneath the condemnation, fear, and ignorance, however, we know at our core that significant change can only happen if we begin with ourselves.

Now is the time to live with certainty; there is no other. This is the time for change and transformation, to discover your true self and to purify and heighten your energy. Anything that you deem meaningful or have longed to do but put off because you were "too busy," pursue now, big or small. This will make you feel productive and create momentum. Now is the perfect time for you to make the decision to begin living intentionally—with purposeful authenticity—and to co-create not only your own life, but also a better world. If we all lived with certainty in alignment with our inspired soul-views, *without question* the world would change for the better. Is there a result that you could hope for that has a higher order? If not now, when?

The Living with Certainty Revolution

Living with Certainty has proven itself to me and to others as a rewarding and powerful way to improve lives irrespective of whom or where you are. The purpose of this text is straightforward—to incite and inspire a worldwide Living with Certainty Revolution that empowers people across the globe to experience their purposeful authenticity and deep-soul joy. We will link together one soul at a time, forming a universal Certainty Chain, creating better lives and a better planet link by link.

If the Living with Certainty life plan resonates with you and you commit to it, thereby transforming your life, then you have everything required to make a positive impact on not only yourself, but on someone else. As you experience more vitality and gratitude, you realize that you have the capacity to serve as a brilliant shining light for others, encouraging and inspiring them to transform their own lives. Remember, the essence of all of our dreams is similar, and through your singular efforts you can have a positive effect on a multitude of others. This is how widespread change happens. Anyone who has experienced the transformational gift of deep-soul joy feels strongly that this knowledge should be shared and feels compelled to teach others who have interest. You will find as you meet others who live with certainty that you sense a significant, empowering energetic connection. As we experience interconnectivity at the soul-level we will begin to respond to each other differently.

Living with Certainty is a process—your awareness, your development, and your becoming are part of this process. As challenging as this new approach may initially seem, the challenges are part and parcel of personal growth and development and you will work through them before you know it. The *Living with Certainty Discovery Guide* will be an invaluable resource to you during your journey. If, however, you're still having trouble, you can reach me through my website (www.LivingwithCertainty.com), and we can discuss how I can personally help you to break through any barriers you are facing.

My driving purpose is to teach the world to Live with Certainty. My journey *can* and *will* make a difference. It's time to stop being too embarrassed or inhibited to talk about spirituality and our souls. The only way to transform the world is one soul at a time. The more we speak of our souls, the less foreign the concept will seem. Let's openly talk about and explore the topics that we *should*—those things that make the world a better place and help to heal people. Join me in the Certainty Chain and together we can change for the better the current trajectory of humanity, learn to experience deep-soul joy, and work to elevate the spiritual energy level across the world through our minds, souls, and loving intentions.

A Final Word

Your success or failure in life does not hinge on one opportunity, or randomly receiving that one big break. You are a brilliant, radiant spiritual being of unlimited love and potential with the hardwired capacity to co-create in every moment the life the universe always intended for you to live. Every day presents you with an opportunity to become and express more of your purposeful authenticity. Believe that the gifts you have can somehow, in some way, *uniquely* serve the world. It's never too late.

You needn't be a yogi, guru, or saint to spread love, peace, and joy, or to play a role in improving life on our planet. With more than six billion people in the world, transforming a fraction of them still amounts to millions of people. My goal is for every person who reads this book to commit to discussing it with others. You then will become a crucial link in the Certainty Chain and in the positive web of energy extending and multiplying from this message.

This is not a trend; rather, this is your new approach to the rest of your life. Make no mistake: If you commit to Living with Certainty, you will discover the best of yourself. Daunting as some of the inner work required may seem, this is the most important work of your life.

And it has a tremendous upside. As each of us begin to grow, heal, put the proper pieces into place, reprioritize, and awaken, one by one we will change the ways of the world. Once this happens, there will never, ever be any going back.

When you live with awareness; when you align with your inspired soul-view; when you feel profound gratitude for every aspect of your life; when you experience more love and compassion than you have ever known; when you experience universal interconnectivity with all people and nature; when you live from a baseline of deep-soul joy; and when your entire life has coalesced into a high-vibrational expression of your purposeful authenticity, *then* you are living with certainty.

Keep inquiring, keep adventuring, and keep pushing the envelope in an effort to understand this mystical, magical universe. Be open to pain, be courageous to progress, be a part of the compassionate energetic revolution for which the world weeps.

> *"May I be a protector to the vulnerable;*
> *A guide to those traveling;*
> *A bridge to those pining;*
> *For the farther shore.*
> *May the suffering of all completely cease.*
> *May I be the healer and the medicine,*
> *Nursing all the sick of this world,*
> *Until everyone is well."*
> —Shantideva

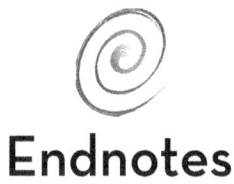

Endnotes

Chapter 2
1. David T. Lykken and Auke Tellegen, "Happiness Is a Stochastic Phenomenon," University of Minnesota, *Psychological Science* Vol.7, No. 3, May 1996. Also available online at http://cogprints.org/767/0/167.pdf.

Chapter 4
2. Das Gesetz der Serie. Ein Lehre von den Wiederholungen im Lebens—und Weltgeschehen. Mit 8 Tafeln und 26. ABB. Deutsche Verlags-Anstalt, Stuttgart/Berlin, 1919.

3. Jim Benton, "The Daytona 500: NASCAR's Super Bowl," Scripps Howard News Service, *The Rocky Mountain News,* February 14, 2008. Also available online at http://www.kypost.com/content/middleblue2/story/The-Daytona-500-NASCARs-Super-Bowl.

Chapter 6
4. Dr. Susan Gregg, *The Complete Idiot's Guide to Spiritual Healing* (Indianapolis: Alpha Books, 2000), 15.

Chapter 9
5. Maharishi Vedic Education Development Corporation, The Transcendental Meditation Program, http://www.tm.org.

Chapter 11
6. Gary Zukav, *The Seat of the Soul* (New York: A Fireside Book by Simon and Schuster, 1989), 98.

Chapter 13
7. John Edward, *One Last Time* (New York: The Berkely Publishing Group, 1998), 44.

Chapter 13

8. Phillip C. McGraw, Ph.D., *The Ultimate Weight Solution: The 7 Keys to Weight Loss Freedom* (New York: Simon & Schuster, Inc./The Free Press) 2003.

9. http://www.worldofquotes.com/author/Doc-Childre/1/index.html.

10. Larry Dossey, M.D., *Healing Words: The Power of Prayer and the Practice of Medicine* (San Francisco: Harper, 1993), 97.

Chapter 14

11. http://www.make-your-goals-happen.com/reticular-activating-system.html.

12. Marianne Williamson, *A Return to Love: Reflections on the Principles of A Course in Miracles* (New York: Harper Collins, 1992) Chapter 7, Section 3.

Chapter 15

13. Tilmann A. Klein, Jane Neumann, Martin Reuter, Jürgen Hennig, D. Yves von Cramon, Markus Ullsperger, "Genetically Determined Differences in Learning from Errors," *Science,* 7 December 2007: Vol. 318. no. 5856, 1642-1645.

14. John Templeton Foundation, http://www.templeton.org/capabilities_2004/pdf/SPIRITUALITY_AND_HEALTH.pdf.

15. http://www.marielhemingway.com/blog/2008

16. Oprah Winfrey, *The Oprah Winfrey Show* (Oprah's Book Club: Sidney Poitier Tribute, March 28, 2007.)

Chapter 16

17. "25 Ways to Show Kids You Care by Building Assets," The Search Institute, Healthy Kids Initiative, 615 First Avenue N.E., Suite 125, Minneapolis, MN 55413, www.search-institute.org

18. http: //www.oprah.com/spirit/Oprah-Interviews-Maria-Shriver/print/1 June 2008 issue of *O, The Oprah Magazine.*

19. www.goop.com/newsletter/30/.

20. United States National Institutes of Health, Office of Medical Applications of Research, "The Health Benefits of Pets," Workshop summary; Bethesda, MD, 1987 Sept. 10–11.

Chapter 17
21. Abraham Joshua Heschel, *Man Is Not Alone: A Philosophy of Religion* (New York: Farrar, Straus, Giroux), 1951.

Chapter 19
22. Deepak Chopra, *The Book of Secrets: Unlock the Hidden Dimensions in Your Life* (New York: Three Rivers Press), 2004.

Chapter 24
23. W. David Hoisington, Ph.D., "Reducing the Negative Effects of Stress: A Workshop for Human Service Professionals." Fall 1998.

Chapter 27
24. Mayo Clinic Staff, "Letting Go of Grudges and Bitterness," http://www.mayoclinic.com/health/forgiveness/mh00131.

Chapter 30
25. Deepak Chopra, *The Book of Secrets: Unlock the Hidden Dimensions in Your Life* (New York: Three Rivers Press), 2004.

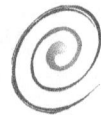

Recommended Reading

Carol Adrienne, *The Purpose of Your Life* (New York: William Morrow & Co., 1998)
Charlene Belitz & Meg Lundstrom, *The Power of Flow/Practical Ways to Transform Your Life with Meaningful Coincidence* (New York: Three Rivers Press, 1998)
Stephan Bodian, *Meditation for Dummies* (Wiley Publishing: 2006)
Gregg Braden, *The Spontaneous Healing of Belief* (Carlsbad, CA: Hay House, Inc., 2008)
Gregg Braden, *The Divine Matrix* (Carlsbad, CA: Hay House, Inc., 2007)
Rhonda Byrne, *The Secret* (New York: Simon & Schuster, Beyond Words Publishing: 2007)
Pema Chodron, *Start Where You Are* (Boston: Shambhala, 2001)
Deepak Chopra, *The Book of Secrets* (New York: Three Rivers Press)
Tony D'Souza and Bud Wonsiewicz, *Discovering Awareness: A Guide to Inner Peace, Strength and Freedom* (Broadway Living Press, 2006)
Dr. Wayne W. Dyer, *Your Ultimate Calling* (Carlsbad, CA: Hay House, Inc., 2008)
———. *The Invisible Force* (Carlsbad, CA: Hay House, Inv., 2007
John Edward, *One Last Time* (New York: Berkley Books, 1999)
Debbie Ford, *The Right Questions: Ten Essential Questions to Guide You to an Extraordinary Life* (San Francisco: Harper Collins, 2004)
Dr. Susan Gregg, *The Complete Idiot's Guide to Spiritual Healing* (Alpha Books: Penguin Group, USA)
Esther and Jerry Hicks, *The Law of Attraction* (Carlsbad, CA: Hay House, Inc., 2007)
Paul Kurtz, *Exuberance/A Philosophy of Happiness* (New York: Prometheus Books, 1977)
Elizabeth Lesser, *The Seeker's Guide: Making Your Life a Spiritual Adventure* (New York: Random House, 1999)
Denise Linn, *The Secret Language Signs: How to Interpret the Coincidences in Your Life* (New York: Random House, 1996
Sadie Nardini, *Road Trip Guide to the Soul: A 9-Step Guide to Reaching Your Inner Self and Revolutionizing Your Life* (New Jersey: John Wiley & Sons, Inc., 2008)

Recommended Reading

Penney Peirce, *Frequency: The Power of Personal Vibration* (New York: Atria Books, 2009)

Mary Anne Radmacher, *Live Boldly* (California: Conari Press, 2008)

Sanaya Roman, *Living with Joy* (California: H. J. Kramer, Inc., 1986)

Marsha Sinetar, *Do What You Love, The Money Will Follow* (New York: Dell Publishing, 1987)

Eckhart Tolle, *A New Earth: Awakening to Your Life's Purpose* (Plume Printing: Penguin Group, USA, 2005)

Patricia Rose Upczak, *Synchronicity Signs & Symbols* (Colorado: Synchronicity Publishing, 2001)

Wallace D. Wattles, *The Science of Getting Rich/Financial Success Through Creative Thought* (New York: Barnes & Noble, 2007 Edition)

Gary Zukav, *Soul to Soul/Communications from the Heart* (New York: Free Press, 2007)

Gary Zukav, *The Seat of the Soul* (New York: Simon & Schuster, 1989)

Jack Canfield and D. D. Watkins, Jack Canfield's *Key to Living the Law of Attraction* (Florida: Health Communications, Inc., 2007)

Marci Shimoff with Carol Kline, *Happy for No Reason* (New York: Free Press, 2008)

Mick Ukleja, Ph.D. and Robert Lorber, Ph.D., *Who Are You and What Do You Want?* (Iowa: Meredith Books, 2008)

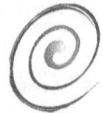

About the Author

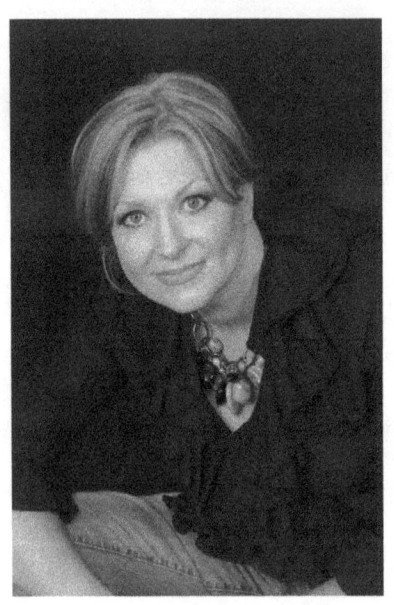

Over many years as a successful senior partner and global practice leader with the world's largest, most prestigious retained executive search firms, Kristi has had the privilege of advising, assessing, coaching, and interviewing thousands of professionals and senior executives, many of whom are the most outwardly successful, accomplished, intelligent, and principled men and women on the planet. These exceptional leaders actively sought her advice. To a person, they all desired more than money from their lives and careers—they wanted creative expression, authenticity, purpose, fulfillment, significance, and joy.

Since Kristi's personal approach to life is to see every facet of the world through a spiritual lens, this perspective ultimately led to the development of her Living with Certainty philosophy. This book represents Kristi's deeply held suppositions gained through her professional career, natural inclination and intuition, research, and personal spiritual experiences.

Kristi is a wife, mom to three small children, author, daughter, sister, and professional woman with a deep desire to teach people how to live with certainty. She lives with deep-soul joy and wishes the same for you.

Kristi welcomes reactions from readers—thoughts, stories, and reflections. Though she is not always able to respond to every email, she enjoys hearing from (and always learns from) her readers. To reach Kristi via email, write her at KristiLeBlanc@LivingwithCertainty.com. For more information on how to Live with Certainty, go to www.LivingwithCertainty.com.

www.ingramcontent.com/pod-product-compliance
Lightning Source LLC
Chambersburg PA
CBHW022108150426
43195CB00008B/315